P9-DTF-783

TREATING DEMENTIA IN CONTEXT

TREATING DEMENTIA IN CONTEXT

A STEP-BY-STEP GUIDE TO WORKING WITH INDIVIDUALS AND FAMILIES

SUSAN M. MCCURRY

CLAUDIA DROSSEL

AMERICAN PSYCHOLOGICAL ASSOCIATION
WASHINGTON, DC

Published by
APA Books
750 First Street, NE
Washington, DC 20002
www.apa.org

To order
APA Order Department
P.O. Box 92984
Washington, DC 20090-2984
Tel: (800) 374-2721; Direct: (202) 336-5510
Fax: (202) 336-5502; TDD/TTY: (202) 336-6123
Online: www.apa.org/books/
E-mail: order@apa.org

In the U.K., Europe, Africa, and the Middle East, copies may be ordered from
American Psychological Association
3 Henrietta Street
Covent Garden, London
WC2E 8LU England

Typeset in Goudy by Circle Graphics, Inc., Columbia, MD

Printer: Maple-Vail Book Manufacturing Group, York, PA
Cover Designer: Minker Design, Sarasota, FL

The opinions and statements published are the responsibility of the authors, and such opinions and statements do not necessarily represent the policies of the American Psychological Association.

Library of Congress Cataloging-in-Publication Data
McCurry, Susan.
 Treating dementia in context : a step-by-step guide to working with individuals and families / Susan M. McCurry and Claudia Drossel. — 1st ed.
    p. ; cm.
 Includes bibliographical references.
 ISBN-13: 978-1-4338-0936-1 (print)
 ISBN-10: 1-4338-0936-2 (print)
 1. Dementia—Treatment. 2. Dementia—Patients—Care. 3. Dementia—Patients—Rehabilitation. I. Drossel, Claudia. II. American Psychological Association. III. Title.
 [DNLM: 1. Dementia—therapy. 2. Caregivers—psychology. 3. Professional-Family Relations. 4. Quality of Life. WM 220]

  RC521.M3898 2011
  616.8'3—dc22
                          2010038520
  616.85'83—dc22
                          2010038515

British Library Cataloguing-in-Publication Data

A CIP record is available from the British Library.

Printed in the United States of America
First Edition

doi:10.1037/12314-000

In the beginning, we don't understand what our client needs, but we have a method for figuring it out.
—*Robert G. Janes, MD, MPH, PS, Psychoanalyst, Seattle, WA*

To Chris and Ian McCurry, who remind me daily that love, laughter, and kindness are at the heart of everything in life that matters.
—*Susan M. McCurry*

To Jane E. Fisher, PhD, who established the Nevada Caregiver Support Center with a vision of restraint-free dementia care, and to the Center's families, from whom we continue to learn.
—*Claudia Drossel*

CONTENTS

FOREWORD

REBECCA G. LOGSDON

As diagnostic procedures have become more sophisticated and treatment options more widely available, medical diagnosis of Alzheimer's disease and other dementias in their earliest stages has become both feasible
and accepted as good clinical practice. Early diagnosis allows treatment to
be started sooner; legal, financial, and residential plans to be developed; and
support services to be identified and mobilized. However, receiving a
dementia diagnosis is a life-altering event for individuals and their families.
Even the best relationships can be challenged as families struggle to cope with
the cognitive, emotional, physical, and social consequences of the disease.
Furthermore, because of the progressive nature of dementia, a diagnosis initiates an ongoing need for education and support that typically continues for
many years.

Most dementia care is, and will continue to be, provided at home by
family members. Typically, one person (either a spouse or an adult child) is
directly responsible for day-to-day care, including assistance with shopping,
cooking, housekeeping, bathing, dressing, and many other tasks. This primary
caregiver also bears the brunt of behavioral changes that occur during the progression of dementia and must be constantly adapting and adjusting to new
and different behaviors. Other family members may (or may not) fulfill specific

roles, such as arranging transportation, providing medical care, going on out-ings, facilitating legal planning, or paying bills. For those who live far away, involvement may consist of telephone calls, financial support, research about services and resources, and periodic visits to provide respite and support for the primary caregiver. While dealing with all these practical challenges and issues, families also are dealing with emotional issues and changes in roles that impact the diagnosed person, the family, and their social networks. For the diagnosed person, loss of activities and independence may trigger depression, anxiety, denial, and other emotional issues. For families, seeing and respond-ing to the changes in their loved one may lead to complex feelings of grief, anger, guilt, and physical exhaustion. Conversely, many diagnosed individu-als and families also identify positive experiences in dealing with the diagno-sis, such as overcoming obstacles, meeting new challenges, and experiencing increased closeness as they work toward common goals.

Compassionate and appropriate dementia care is challenging and requires knowledge and skills that are unique to each individual and family. The good news is that the requisite skills can be learned and developed grad-ually over the course of the caregiving career. As described in this volume, a good foundation requires an understanding of cognitive impairment and its impact on both behavioral and emotional functioning of the affected indi-vidual. This understanding leads to realistic expectations, good communica-tion skills, and the ability to empathize with the diagnosed family member. In time, problems that once seemed insurmountable become manageable, as the caregiver learns a framework for objectively analyzing behaviors and gains the skills to develop and implement plans to reduce disturbing behaviors and to increase pleasant, meaningful activities. As caregivers are able to interact positively with the person with dementia, they can also learn self-care skills that will help them navigate the long, sometimes exhausting, but ultimately rewarding process of "caregiver-hood."

This volume is based on a solid research foundation, a vast amount of practical clinical experience, and, most important, a deep and abiding sense of compassion and respect for individuals and families affected by dementia. Drs. McCurry and Drossel have provided an invaluable resource for psychol-ogists, social workers, counselors, nurses, and others who form the professional network that supports these individuals and families. Using the framework of the DANCE of dementia care and giving detailed and practical examples of how to apply behavioral problem-solving strategies to a wide variety of issues that occur throughout the course of dementia, clinicians will learn skills that can be applied with widely divergent individuals and families at any stage of their caregiving careers. The authors focus on evidence-based treatment approaches supported by rigorous scientific research and provide guidelines for choosing among different treatment alternatives. They also provide realistic and engaging examples of how these approaches can be used in a compassionate and effective way.

In dementia care, maintaining quality of life for both the diagnosed person and the family caregiver requires a unique and ever-changing combination of problem-solving skills, creativity, flexibility, and acceptance. Health care professionals, educators, and counselors can be instrumental in assisting families as they deal with changing roles and responsibilities and in facilitating difficult decisions that must be made along the way. This book is a guide that clinicians will reach for over and over for education, ideas, and examples of how to help caregivers deal with difficult problems while maintaining their own mental and physical health.

ACKNOWLEDGMENTS

Throughout our careers and over the course of this project, we have been fortunate to have worked with and learned from many people who are experts in the fields of gerontology and behavioral psychology. In particular, we would like to thank the following individuals for sharing their time, wisdom, mentorship, clinical skills, research experiences, and critical feedback:

Rebecca G. Logsdon, Linda Teri, and Michael Vitiello, University of Washington

Eric B. Larson, Group Health Research Institute

William C. Follette, Steven S. Graybar, Steven C. Hayes, and Duane L. Varble, University of Nevada, Reno

Barry D. Lebowitz and Sonia Ancoli-Israel, University of California, San Diego; George T. Niederehe, National Institute of Mental Health; Charles F. Reynolds III, University of Pittsburgh; and all the faculty at the NIMH/AAGP Summer Research Institute in Geriatric Psychiatry

James D. Bowen, Wayne C. McCormick, Meredith Pfanschmidt, Sheila O'Connell, and "the ACT gang" at the University of Washington and Group Health Research Institute

Amy Moore, June Van Leynseele, and the research team at the University of
Washington Northwest Research Group on Aging, Seattle, Washington
Philip Hineline and Tim Shipley, Temple University, Philadelphia, Penn-
sylvania

We would also like to thank Susan Reynolds, senior acquisitions editor
at APA books, who first approached us about writing this book and continued
to offer encouragement, invaluable editorial advice, and support throughout
its conception and birth.

Last, we hold close to our hearts the many persons with dementia and
their caregivers who have shared their lives with us. This book would not
have been possible without the individuals whose stories grace these pages.
In gratitude to their generosity, we have taken care to protect their identity
by changing not only names and demographic information but also details
of problems, relationships, and life circumstances. Frequently, we weaved
together multiple lives to illustrate a point. If you believe you recognize a
friend, neighbor, or family member, it is only because the challenges, sorrows,
and triumphs described in this book are universal to the world of individuals
with dementia and their caregivers.

TREATING DEMENTIA IN CONTEXT

INTRODUCTION

SUSAN M. McCURRY

My family often spends the Fourth of July holiday with friends at their beach house on Guemas Island in Washington. We take long walks along the island's lovely shore, which is covered with pebbles and rocks of all sizes, shapes, and colors. I love collecting rocks and always come home with my pockets full of those that catch my fancy. My friend, however, is usually hunting for agates—beautiful, tiny, golden-clear crystals that sparkle in the sun as one walks by. Since her childhood growing up on this beach, she has found hundreds, if not thousands, of these tiny jewels, which she keeps in an enormous jar. In contrast, over the years I had been visiting, I had never found an agate. Searching the ground as I strolled along, I would zero in on rocks of certain sizes, bright colors, or unusual shapes or patterns. The unassuming, tiny agates were too subtle for me and were lost in the distractingly diverse topography of the beach debris all around them. My eyes could only see what they were accustomed to seeing.

On our most recent trip it occurred to me that my inability to find agates was a metaphor for dementia care. We tend to see in our family members and loved ones, in our clients, even in ourselves, only what we expect and are looking for. As long as situations are static, seeing only what is familiar can be a highly successful strategy. A diagnosis of progressive dementia, however,

3

slowly alters self-expression and the rules of interpersonal engagement. One person who looks the same externally is starting to experience the world in a vastly unfamiliar way but may not be able to share with us in words the changes that are occurring. Another person who is behaving quite differently may be oblivious to the fact that anything is the matter and resists our efforts to tell them otherwise.

This book is an attempt to help you track the unexpected changes and to start to see persons with dementia differently. We would like you to look at them with new eyes, in the midst of all the hustle and bustle of the health care professional's busy world, and to learn to recognize subtle signs that reveal what people with dementia need and who they are. We want to help you see the precious jewels of selfhood that are preserved in every individual with dementia, no matter how advanced their disease or how distracted you may become dealing with surprising behaviors.

This book is designed to be of use to health care professionals with various clinical backgrounds and levels of experience with dementia. Our emphasis is problem oriented, applied, and practical: How do you go about preventing or reducing the emotional and behavioral changes that are so common in persons with dementia? To answer this question and to provide you with a range of interventions, we consider the many physical, environmental, interpersonal, and historical factors that influence behavior. We wrote the book thinking of trainees and colleagues who have consulted with us about their cognitively impaired clients' difficulties; what did these colleagues need to know about the person with dementia to increase the likelihood that their treatment recommendations would be appropriate for the situation, understood by the client or caregiver(s), properly implemented and monitored, and also be maximally effective?

Our specialty is the prevention or reduction of behavioral and affective changes by nonpharmacological means. In this book, we do not discuss specific pharmacological treatments, but we recognize that many of your clients will be taking one or more psychotropic or cognitive function enhancing medications. Thus, we address the use of these medications generally—particularly with regard to their potential side effect risks—and recommend that you consult with a geriatric psychiatrist or pharmacist in evaluating their role in your clients' care. Similarly, although we do not discuss the epidemiology of cognitive decline, anatomical or biochemical pathology, or neuropsychological assessment procedures, proper diagnosis and neurophysiological knowledge are important. We strongly recommend you seek out opportunities to learn more from specialists in these areas.

The book is laid out in three parts. The first part, "Setting the Stage," gives the reader an overview of what dementia is and how we are going to approach understanding the context in which behavior changes occur. Chapter 1 describes the most common cognitive and behavioral symptoms of dementia, with an emphasis on how these symptoms affect clients' view of themselves and the world. We have written this chapter to provide a novice health care practitioner or person new to working with cognitively impaired individuals key information about dementia syndromes and to give more advanced practitioners new insights into what the cognitive, affective, and behavioral symptoms of dementia may be communicating about the client seeking help. In Chapter 2, we describe the contextual approach to dementia care that we use for conceptualizing and developing treatment plans with our clients. In this chapter, you will learn basic behavior analytic terms, illustrated with clinical examples and presented in language that make them accessible to psychologists and non-psychologists alike.

Part II describes the actual process of working with cognitively impaired clients across the spectrum of care. We organized this section of the book around the acronym DANCE, which is described in Chapter 3. The DANCE acronym has proved to be a useful heuristic for helping family caregivers remember a set of simple principles associated with creative, compassionate dementia care. We follow several typical case examples throughout Part II and introduce many clinical vignettes to illustrate how the contextual model can be used to develop and monitor collaborative treatment plans with your clients. Much of the material in this section is vitally important to the real clients we serve, but it is not often talked about in dementia care books. For example, Chapter 4 describes the process of establishing rapport and evaluating consent to treatment with cognitively impaired individuals. Chapter 5 talks about the most common medical comorbidities that evoke mood and behavior changes, including adverse effects of medication. In Chapter 6, we discuss the importance of helping caregivers maintain or reestablish respectful and intimate connections with spouses, parents, friends, or clients who have dementia. Chapter 7 describes why nonpharmacological interventions are considered the first line of treatment for managing mood and behavior changes in dementia. We discuss how the contextual model of dementia care is similar to, and different from, other evidence-based treatments and how these other treatments can inform your problem solving around common symptoms such as depression, agitation and aggression, wandering and circadian rhythm disturbances, and erroneous beliefs and accusatory behaviors. Last, in Chapter 8, we emphasize the importance and possibility of helping your clients with dementia and their caregivers experience and maintain a rich quality of life despite disease progression and changing symptom patterns. Note that the names and details in all cases discussed have been changed to protect the anonymity of the clients.

The closing part of the book, Part III, is a reminder of the many things that you, the health care professional, can gain from your work with cognitively impaired individuals. As noted in Chapter 9, those of us who work with persons with dementia learn something new every day from our clients, and we are better people for it. One of our hopes for this book is that it will encourage and inspire more health care professionals to move into clinical work with older adults, which will mean serving persons at all stages of cognitive function. Throughout the book, we have inserted notations that will provide the interested reader with additional scientific references and details regarding various topics of interest. Several appendices are also included at the end. These provide you with lists of standardized cognitive, functional, and behavioral assessment instruments and their source citations (Appendix A), a blank behavioral tracking form that you can modify and use in your own practices (Appendix B), a sample case report illustrating how a complete case might treated and summarized (Appendix C), and lists of relevant and interesting aging and dementia care resources (Appendix D).

In sum, we have tried to give you everything you need to be a more creative and effective provider in your work with cognitively impaired individuals. Throughout the text, we remind our readers repeatedly: "We can do more than we think we can to help persons with dementia and their caregivers."

Last Fourth of July, for the first time, I found an agate. My friend's gentle coaching, my desire to find one of these hidden treasures, and simple practice is teaching me to see the world differently. We hope this book can do the same for you.

I

SETTING THE STAGE

1

MAKING SENSE OF THE DIAGNOSIS

If you are reading this book, chances are that you are someone who has regular contact with older adults and who cares deeply about helping them maintain their independence, dignity, and quality of life for as long as possible. Is that not what we all want for our loved ones—and for ourselves as we age? Many people, however, feel that a diagnosis of Alzheimer's disease or some other form of dementia destroys all hope for a maintained quality of life in the future. If this has been your view of dementia, then we hope, through this book, to convince you otherwise. Although dementia, like any chronic disease, certainly alters the direction a life will take, for much of its course the signs and symptoms of disease can be managed in ways that respect a person's individuality, preferences, and sense of self. But those with dementia cannot do it alone. They need our help to maintain a life of safety, dignity, and enrichment. Whatever your professional background or interest in dementia, this book will teach you the skills you need to be a person who can provide such support.

In this chapter, we set the stage by inviting you to think about how dementia affects your clients from their point of view and how the symptoms of dementia affect a person's ability to maintain a sense of purpose and identity in the world. Many of the emotional and behavioral changes that emerge when somebody experiences increasing difficulties communicating, problem

9

solving, or remembering make sense in the context of the person's historical and current life circumstances. We also discuss how dementia-related work can affect your own point of view and the personal and professional skills that you will find stimulated and enriched from working with cognitively impaired individuals. The term *dementia care* implies that the relationship between individuals with dementia and their family members or health care workers is unidirectional: The person with dementia receives help, and the other person (the caregiver) offers assistance and aid. However, in reality it is more the case that both sides can benefit from and be changed by traveling this journey together. Effective dementia care is deeply compassionate work that invites us to build genuine relationships with our clients and, in the process, to learn much about ourselves.

WHAT IS DEMENTIA?

The term *dementia* refers to both a clinical syndrome—defined by criteria outlined in diagnostic manuals—and the symptoms associated with certain detectable neuropathological changes. Dementia as a clinical syndrome is broadly defined by three criteria: (a) multiple deficits in cognitive skills, (b) a notable decline from previous skill levels, and (c) a significant disruption of daily routines and common activities. The observed deficits, the decline, and the disruption of daily functioning must be determined to be irreversible and not attributable to acute, treatable conditions with abrupt onset, such as medical illnesses or noxious injury, medication side effects, or substance intoxication (*delirium*). According to these three general criteria, approximately 75% to 84% of the population will develop some type of dementia before they die. If you work with older adults, the chances are excellent that you will encounter persons who meet the clinical criteria for dementia.

As a clinical syndrome, dementia can be quite varied in its presentation. When Alois Alzheimer in 1906 described his first case of "presenile dementia" in a 51-year-old woman,[1] he mistakenly assumed that the characteristic brain pathology he was seeing was only found in younger individuals and that all late-life cognitive decline was caused by arteriosclerosis. Since then, science has made monumental strides in the development of diagnostic criteria that link specific clusters of cognitive symptoms to specific types of neurological disease. Although Alzheimer's disease is the most common form of dementia, it is now clear there are over 70 distinct organic disorders that

---

[1]Alois Alzheimer first reported the case of 51-year-old Frau Auguste D. at the meeting of South–West Germany psychiatrists in November 1906, in Tübingen, Germany (Bick, 1999).

cause dementia (Katzman, 2002), and it is not rare for an older adult to be afflicted with more than one. In this book we will not review the standard medical procedures for making a dementia diagnosis or for differentiating dementia subtypes because these are described well elsewhere.[2] However, it is important to understand that the particular type and location of brain pathology associated with your clients' diagnosis create the context from which behavioral challenges arise, and these biological contributions increasingly influence behavior as the disease progresses. Because particular neurodegenerative diseases may bring about characteristic patterns of novel behaviors, when working with individuals with dementia knowledge about the specific type of diagnosed dementia is useful (see Table 1.1). We should also note that it is always important to consider whether delirium—including medication side effects—might be contributing to your client's behavioral symptoms.[3] In Chapter 5, we spend a great deal of time discussing how dementia and delirium interact to create behavior changes in cognitively impaired individuals.

HOW DEMENTIA AFFECTS YOUR CLIENTS

As important as a dementia diagnosis is to predicting behavioral symptoms, it is not the whole story. Within any given disease subtype, a person's individual behavioral patterns can be quite idiosyncratic. Thus, the first step to effective dementia care is trying to understand the unique experience of your client: what particular symptoms he or she has and how these symptoms are impacting the quality of life. Exhibit 1.1 summarizes the various dementia-related behavioral symptoms to consider, which are described in greater detail next.

Memory

Although not every cognitively impaired individual has significant memory decline, diagnostic criteria have traditionally emphasized the importance of memory disturbances. The current version of the *Diagnostic and Statistical*

---

[2]Two excellent descriptions of the dementia diagnostic process, including a review of cognitive screening instruments most widely used in primary care and issues related to differential diagnoses, can be found in Holsinger, Deveau, Boustani, and Williams (2007) and Ross and Bowen (2002). Of related interest is the issue of how a dementia diagnosis should be disclosed to a client. For discussion of the factors that contribute to effective disclosure, see Lecouturier et al. (2008). For an interesting analysis of the functional utility of the term *dementia* as a diagnostic classification, see Kurz and Lautenschlager (2010).
[3]A 2006 special issue of *Journal of Gerontology: Medical Sciences* presented a series of articles relevant to understanding the interrelationship of dementia and delirium, introduced nicely by Inouye and Ferrucci (2006).

TABLE 1.1
Distinctive Cognitive–Behavioral Features of Disorders That Lead to Dementia or Dementia-Related Changes

Organic condition	Features	Additional information
	Cerebral disorders	
Alzheimer's disease	Memory problems are most prominent early symptom, with additional problems including impaired language (aphasia), motor and visuospatial difficulties, disorientation, problems with simple math (acalculia).	Most common dementia; slowly progressing except in more rare autosomal dominant (usually early onset) forms; contextual cues generally do not facilitate remembering
Frontotemporal dementias	Tendency to respond impulsively, failure to self-monitor performance, memory loss, pronounced difficulty in executive functioning and language production (e.g., inability to repeat, stereotyped utterances, reduced speech)	Slowly progressing; contextual cues often facilitate remembering; also known as Pick's disease, dementia of the frontal type, frontal lobe dementia of the non-Alzheimer's type, frontotemporal lobar degeneration, semantic dementia, and progressive nonfluent aphasia
Lewy bodies	Prominent deficits on tests of attention, executive function, and visuospatial ability; fluctuating cognition with pronounced variations in attention and alertness; well-formed and detailed visual hallucinations; parkinsonism physical signs	Third most common dementia subtype; slowly progressing; REM sleep behavior disorder and severe neuroleptic sensitivity might be suggestive of Lewy bodies disease.
Parkinson's disease	Resting tremor; rigidity; slowness in movement (bradykinesia); postural instability; impairment in attention, memory, executive and visuospatial functions; visual hallucinations; apathy	Slowly progressing; dementia occurs in approximately 30% of Parkinson's disease cases; main pathological correlate is Lewy body-type degeneration.
Prion diseases (e.g., Creutzfeldt-Jakob)	Muscular twitching and spasms (myoclonus), incoordination (ataxia), rigidity, prominent memory loss, behavioral changes	Rare; rapidly progressing dementia

TABLE 1.1
Distinctive Cognitive–Behavioral Features of Disorders That Lead to
Dementia or Dementia-Related Changes   *(Continued)*

Organic condition	Features	Additional information
Normal pressure hydrocephalus	Preceded by gait disorder and incontinence; slowed processing speed; apathy; later global cognitive dysfunction, including memory loss	Aphasia and object recognition (agnosia) deficits are rare.
Trauma	Headache, variable extrapyramidal signs (e.g., restlessness, movement and muscle tension disorders)	Aphasia is rare.
	Systemic disorders	
Vascular disorders	Focal neurological signs and symptoms; laboratory evidence of cerebrovascular disease; temporal relationship of stroke and dementia; decline in memory, executive functioning, social functioning, language, and muscle control	Second most common dementia subtype, particularly co-occurring with Alzheimer's disease (mixed dementia); abrupt onset; stepwise deterioration; somatic complaints
Cardiogenic dementia	Early loss of executive functioning, slowed fine motor speed, loss of memory and motor functioning	Related to anoxia or hypoxia (subnormal levels of oxygen to the tissues or brain)
Pulmonary disease	Impaired abstract reasoning, flexible thinking, memory, and performance speed	Related to hypoxia or hypercapnia (CO_2 elevations)
Cancer (brain tumors)	Prominent slowing in processing speed, apathy, impaired concentration, headache, seizures, focal sensorimotor disturbances	Memory loss, aphasia, or agnosia depending on localization of tumor
Infection (e.g., AIDS, neurosyphilis)	Sensory and memory loss, psychomotor retardation, extrapyramidal signs, psychosis	

(continues)

TABLE 1.1
Distinctive Cognitive–Behavioral Features of Disorders That Lead to Dementia or Dementia-Related Changes *(Continued)*

Organic condition	Features	Additional information
	Metabolic disorders	
Alcoholic dementia	Memory loss prominent, rhythmical oscillations of the eyeballs (nystagmus), gait ataxia	
Hypothyroidism	Hair loss, skin changes, headache, hearing loss, tinnitus, vertigo, ataxia, delayed relaxation of tendon reflexes	
Vitamin B_{12} deficiency	Macrocytic anemia, low serum vitamin B_{12} level, psychosis, sensory disturbance, spastic paraparesis (mild paralysis)	
	Organ failure	
Dialysis dementia	Speech articulation problems (dysarthria), myoclonus, seizures	Rare; mean survival is 6 months
Hepatocerebral degeneration	Fluctuating mental status, dysarthria, extrapyramidal signs, memory loss, impaired attention and concentration, abnormal hepatic blood chemistries	Progressive over 1–9 years

Note. This table only summarizes major categories of more common dementia syndromes found in older adults. It is designed to illustrate the complexities of different dementia presentations and should not be considered an exhaustive list of subtypes and symptoms. Data from Emre et al. (2007); Festa and Lazar (2009); Greenberg, Aminoff, and Simon (2002); Kukull and Bowen (2009); Hutchinson and Mathias (2007).

EXHIBIT 1.1
Symptoms Associated With Dementia

Memory
  Recent
  Remote
Communication (aphasia)
Intentional activity (apraxia)
Recognition (agnosia)
Executive function
  Judgment
  Problem solving
  Behavior initiation and cessation
  Abstract reasoning

Orientation
Attention and concentration
Perception
  Visual
  Auditory
  Tactile, olfactory, gustatory
Motor coordination
Emotional and behavioral
  Personality

Note. There are a growing number of instruments appropriate for assessing cognitive, functional, affective, and behavioral changes in persons with dementia and their family caregivers, including many neuropsychological measures normed for older adults. A full discussion of these is beyond the scope of this book. However, we have provided a list of the most common screening instruments used in clinical practice, with key reference citations, in Appendix A.

Manual of Mental Disorders (4th ed., text rev.; *DSM–IV–TR;* American Psychiatric Association, 2000) requires a person to have multiple cognitive deficits, including memory problems plus at least one other symptom, to receive a dementia diagnosis. The nature of the memory problem can vary widely from person to person, particularly early in the disease. It is not unusual for someone to remember past events, such as childhood activities, but not what was served for lunch a few hours ago. A client may draw a blank when asked to describe a current event in the news but can easily repeat stories he or she has told frequently in the past, just as you or I may retell a joke or use an example that has previously swayed an audience, earned us smiles or laughter, or generated understanding. As the disease progresses, fluent speech episodes may become limited to one or two favorite topics, such as how much a person loves her children or how he met his wife.

Particularly early on, the care recipient's inconsistent memory lapses are confusing; the person with dementia may forget seemingly "easy" information, such as an address, telephone number, or items on a shopping list, yet recall details about distant events, especially those that had high emotional significance, such as the death of a spouse or attendance at a wedding. The differing degrees to which emotional versus factual information or overlearned versus new events are remembered make memory seem unpredictable. A person may not be able to remember the names of loved ones anymore (explicit or overt memory) but may still know that they are familiar. (When we asked one care recipient for his wife's name, he answered, "Love.") Research using measures of skin conductance has shown that the ability to state a name and the ability to nonverbally recognize a face are two different skills,[4] so the person who does not remember a loved one's name may still have a strong sense of intimacy and connection.

Episodic or gradually increasing short-term memory problems can generate considerable anxiety in our clients and frustration for those around them. Forgotten conversations with loved ones may lead to feelings of loneliness and isolation and create misunderstandings with important people in our clients' lives. A woman who insists she never received a notice about an overdue bill is furious when her credit card is cancelled and, understandably, accuses the company of foul play. Household and personal objects, or even other people, seem to disappear and reappear in an unpredictable fashion, causing a grandfather to accuse his housekeeper of theft or his wife of having

---

[4]Studies abound that demonstrate "covert" cognitive ability when "expressive" and "overt" verbal knowledge are lacking, and have a long tradition. Sources for consideration of this issue include Tranel and Damasio (1985) for facial recognition without awareness, Hefferline and Perrera (1963) for being able to discern a situation while being unable to describe it, Bechara et al. (1995) for autonomic or classical conditioning without awareness, and Eldridge, Masterman, and Knowlton (2002) for implicit habit learning in Alzheimer's disease.

an affair. Loved ones try to explain the facts, and arguments follow because the person denies being forgetful or fills in memory gaps with "best guess" information that seems to the observer to be blatant lies (confabulation). Loss of one's memories and the associated altered social relationships challenge a person's concept of self and his or her role identity. For some people this is incredibly painful and frightening.

Communication (Aphasia)

As dementia progresses, many individuals experience a wide variety of communicative difficulties. They may not be able to find words, comprehend complex statements, or express abstract ideas. Speaking errors are common (e.g., "My daughter was petting her cap" instead of "cat"). Many people lose their ability to share actual past and current events with a listener, and speech may become increasingly abstract, metaphorical, or disjointed (e.g., "The hairs on my head are fighting," rather than, "I have a headache"). Other people retain excellent social conversational skills, but the content of their conversation is vague or irrelevant to what is going on around them. Even when physical speech is seemingly unimpeded, individuals may lose their ability to explain their behavioral or emotional reactions; for example, a person with dementia may not be able to explain, "I become scared when I'm home alone" or tell you how he or she is physically feeling ("I'm nauseated" or "I have a pain in my side"). The ability to follow multiple speakers may also diminish, causing social events to become overwhelming and anxiety-producing activities. However, it is important to note that despite these difficulties, persons with dementia still want and need to communicate with those around them and to do so verbally. Like all human beings regardless of dementia diagnosis, difficulty comprehending others or expressing oneself can lead to feelings of frustration, verbal or physical aggression, or depression and withdrawal.

Performing Previously Learned Tasks (Apraxia)

Persons with dementia who have physiologically intact motor and sensory function may hear and repeat back instructions to perform some task, such as snapping their fingers or clapping their hands, but then be unable to perform the requested activity. Some individuals not only lose the ability to perform or pantomime actions, but they may also not even be able to fathom trying to execute an action in a goal-directed way. Some behavior that is labeled as "lack of motivation" may, in fact, reflect an inability to initiate or complete activities (e.g., washing the dishes, putting pants on properly) that for many years were second nature.

Recognizing Objects and People (Agnosia)

Individuals with dementia may lose their ability to recognize common objects or engage in goal-directed behavior with respect to them, despite intact visual acuity. A person may, for example, be led to the restroom after he has indicated an urge to urinate but act "lost" in the bathroom because he fails to recognize the toilet. Alternatively, he may be discovered toileting in a houseplant that appeared to him to be a suitable receptacle. People may fail to recognize their loved ones or their own mirror image and become frightened enough to strike out and injure themselves or those around them. People may also mistake one person for another: A grown daughter becomes "mother," a great-grandson a "baby brother" from the distant past, or a female paid caregiver "my wife."

Executive Functioning

The ability to perform multistep problem-solving and abstraction tasks, such as solving mathematical problems, may be impaired. Individuals seem not to be able to "talk themselves through" a problem or to strategize toward a solution, making simple decisions such as what to wear or what to choose from a restaurant menu overwhelming. Concomitantly, they may not be able to shift their behavior to new strategies and so perseverate in repetitive yet ineffective actions. Many of the more sensational behaviors associated with dementia are due to a deterioration in executive function: the banker who loses his savings entering magazine sweepstakes, the woman who sells her house to a dishonest neighbor for a pittance, the grandfather who runs away with a pole dancer 50 years his junior, the grandmother who loudly comments in church about how fat the choir director has become. As organizational and planning skills deteriorate, behavior may become more impulsive and uncharacteristic of the individual's previous patterns.

Orienting

The most common symptom of disorientation is the inability to state the correct date and time. Often, orientation to place or purpose is also disrupted. A woman insists that she wants to "go home" although she is in the same house she has occupied for decades. Time can be quite fluid in persons with dementia, who sometimes react to persons and situations with routines of the past: getting up and dressing as if to go to work, tending to a grandchild's baby doll as if it were a real infant, retelling remote happenings as current events. As dementia progresses, difficulties with place-finding extend from losing one's way while driving on a highway to not being able to find the bathroom at home. At the end of a visit to your office, a client may identify you as her realtor because you had been speaking to her about residential long-term care arrangements. The inability to orient, particularly in combination with declining executive function, puts individuals with dementia at high risk of personal danger or distress (e.g., from getting lost on a short walk) and exploitation by unscrupulous individuals.

Attention and Concentration

Individuals with dementia become increasingly sensitive to distraction and unable to sustain engagement with tasks requiring an extended attention span. Noisy activity rooms, physical clutter, a television playing in the background, or even the everyday bustle of a typical family household can be distracting to someone with cognitive impairment. Functional implications for poor attention include clients' need for frequent prompting and redirection to tasks at hand, such as finishing a meal, getting dressed, or staying seated during church services. Poor concentration also contributes to the challenges many caregivers face finding pleasant activities during the day to keep persons with dementia awake, busy, and out of trouble.

Perceptual Changes

In the past decade, dementia-related decrements in sensory perception, including those that occur in the apparent absence of anatomical changes to peripheral sensory pathways, have received increasing attention.[5] Changes in taste and smell may affect appetite and lead to significant weight gain or loss, because some persons lose interest in eating, develop particular food aversions, or develop cravings, most commonly for sweets. Changes in tactile sense perception have resulted in persons failing to notice when they were injured or accidentally scalding themselves because they could not correctly distinguish unsafe water temperatures. Acute hearing loss may lead to suspiciousness that one is being excluded or talked about. Central auditory dysfunction (i.e., difficulty understanding speech in the presence of background noise) can also affect the ability of even otherwise presymptomatic individuals to follow a conversation in the midst of competing conversations, making it difficult to stay engaged in family or social gatherings. Damage to visual path-

---

[5]Much has been written about the importance of sensory changes as an early diagnostic marker for Alzheimer's disease; for examples, see Devanand et al. (2000); Gates, Anderson, Feeney, McCurry, and Larson (2008); Graves et al., (1999); Müller, Richter, Weisbrod, and Klingberg, (1992); Rizzo, Anderson, Dawson, and Nawrot (2000); and Tippett and Sergio (2006). Although all sensory changes also have functional implications, those related to hearing and vision have the most profound impact on everyday life and should always be considered as part of a contextual analysis of behavior changes in dementia.

ways has particular significance for many of the cognitive performance deficits described earlier. Attention, reading, orientation (i.e., way-finding and localization), and recognition may be diminished as a result of deficits in spatial contrast sensitivity, color perception, stereopsis, and motion perception, including the perception of self-motion.

It is important for us as health care providers to question whether individuals with dementia are experiencing the world as we do, because their perceptions can affect their safety and ability to follow through with treatment recommendations. For example, you may observe a person in your office attempting to step up and over textual gradients in floor covering (e.g., distinct carpet patterns, transitions from carpet to linoleum). Those who are not able to master visuospatial construction tasks (e.g., drawing a clock, a cube, or other stimulus items from dementia rating instruments) may be at risk while driving and incur an increased risk of falls. Pronounced visual disturbances are also common in some forms of dementia, such as dementia with Lewy bodies. Hallucinations often consist of movement perceived "out of the corner of one's eye." Although distressing to caregivers, affected individuals may be simply surprised or briefly wonder about their experience but may not show signs of upset. Instead, they may ask for corroboration of the experience (e.g., "Hey, did you see the little bats flying by?") or engage otherwise in attempts to make sense of unusual visions. For example, if a person has a history of religious faith or spirituality, he or she may relate these perceptual experiences to spirits or ghosts of deceased loved ones and talk about their presence. Assessment of hallucinations must include an evaluation of the person's and the caregiver's response to the experience.

Motor and Coordination Changes

Damage to motor pathways are predominant in some dementias, such as dementia associated with Parkinson's or Huntington's disease and in advanced Alzheimer's disease. When movement occurs, it may be disrupted, jerky, or uncoordinated. Gait disturbances or tremors can be present, and even an overlearned movement, such as signing one's name, may be executed with difficulty only. Such motor and coordination challenges are sometimes highly visible to other individuals and may negatively impact a person's self-image and personal esteem. Movement disorders can also interfere with individuals' ability to hold utensils or a coffee cup at mealtime, safely navigate stairs, shave, tie shoelaces, or engage in any number of motor skills essential to hobbies and recreational activities that may have in the past contributed greatly to a person's quality of life. Many individuals with dementia are unaware of the extent of their difficulties, which raises the specter of real safety concerns for clients who continue to drive, operate power tools, cook, hunt with loaded guns, climb on their rooftops to clean the gutters, or perform any of an endless number of daily activities that can be dangerous to someone without fully functional motor control.

Motivational Changes

Apathy, or significantly diminished interest in previously meaningful or pleasurable activities, may accompany progressive cognitive decline and can be predictive of potential changes in motor functioning. Caregivers often complain that their loved ones, who previously enjoyed social events and were generally curious and interested in their surroundings, now seem content to sit in their favorite chair for hours. Some caregivers may be frustrated or even angered by the lack of motivation, interpreting it as laziness. It is important to evaluate whether such indifference to activity is due to depression, which is often highly treatable, or to other cognitive, perceptual, or motor changes that may need to be more directly managed.

Emotional and Behavioral Changes

Emotional and behavioral changes are ubiquitous when a person experiences a progressive decline in multiple cognitive domains, sensory perception, and motor functioning. Up to 80% of individuals with progressive cognitive decline exhibit emotional and behavioral symptoms, such as fear and anxiety, depression and social withdrawal, restlessness, suspicion and paranoia, or self-protective behaviors (e.g., resistance to personal care; Lyketsos et al., 2002). These unexpected and distressing changes in a person's mood, personality, and behavior place a heavy burden on family relationships and are more highly correlated with caregiver distress and care recipient institutionalization than are many other cognitive symptoms. Living with someone who is physically threatening, who does not sleep, or who is too frightened to let you leave his or her sight is much more difficult than reminding him or her what day it is or what he or she had for lunch.

Much of this book will focus on these emotional and behavioral changes, including how to systematically assess them and intervene. As health care providers, it is our task to help individuals with dementia and their families master unusually taxing and extraordinary circumstances, and nonpharmacological interventions are the first-line, recommended way to do this. An important guiding principle is that the more you know about the person having problems and his or her strengths and weaknesses and tendencies, the more helpful you can be. Although nothing in an individual's history has explicitly prepared him or her to cope with the gravity and severity of creeping functional impairment and the concurrent loss of communicative abilities, many individuals with dementia not only cope but also remain connected within meaningful relationships till the end. In the process of helping clients maintain important life connections in the face of progressive neurodegenerative decline, we can learn a great deal about the courage and resilience of the human spirit and also much about ourselves.

A LOOK AHEAD

We have seen in this chapter that dementia is like a tricky puzzle: It has many different causes and many different appearances that shift and change in often unexpected ways. We, as health care providers, are often as mystified as our clients about where to begin and what to do next. In this book, we illustrate for you, step-by-step, how to develop a behavioral health care plan. The approach we use is evidence based but also clinically flexible and able to be adapted to your particular health care practice needs. With four unfolding clinical examples, we show you how to use the *contextual model of dementia care* to develop personalized treatments that fit a person's unique history and current social, cultural, and physiological circumstances. We teach you to connect with your cognitively impaired clients and help you identify comorbid conditions that complicate diagnosis and treatment. We give you tools for building collaborative relationships with caregivers and professional colleagues and introduce you to the psychosocial treatment literature specific to dementia. We show you that you can do more for individuals with dementia and their families than you might think, by turning the uniquely personal, intimate, and relational aspects of dementia into pivotal points of intervention for real emotional and behavioral change.

2

THE CONTEXTUAL MODEL
OF DEMENTIA CARE

In the next several chapters, we introduce you to specific cases that will prepare you to begin working with persons with dementia and their families. But first, we would like to tell you about our approach to dementia care, particularly our conceptualization of why each individual client develops very different and personal patterns of affective, cognitive, and behavioral changes in response to a neurodegenerative disorder. Health care professionals working with dementia clients come from diverse training backgrounds. They vary in how much experience and contact they have with cognitively impaired individuals and in how they interpret dementia-related behaviors. This diversity enriches our practice. It allows us to see clients from different perspectives and to bring different intervention strengths to the table. Nevertheless, it is easier to proceed in a systematic fashion and communicate our different viewpoints if we have a coherent model to describe the client's situation and needs, and to develop an effective care plan. In this chapter, we introduce readers to the contextual model that we use in our clinical practices to guide this information-gathering process.

DEMENTIA AFFECTS EVERYONE DIFFERENTLY

As briefly mentioned in the previous chapter, the emotional and behavioral changes associated with a dementing illness are not caused solely by neurodegenerative changes to the brain. Rather, each man or woman's personal *context*—his or her personality and history of experiences, culture, psychosocial environment, and physical and emotional health—contributes to the particular symptoms he or she will experience. Sir William Osler (1849–1919), a Canadian physician, noted, "Variability is the law of life, and as no two faces are the same, so no two bodies are alike, and no two individuals react alike and behave alike under the abnormal conditions which we know as disease" (Osler, 1932, p. 331). So, too, no two clients with dementia are alike; because everybody is unique, the effects of neurodegenerative diseases on each person will also be personal and highly individualized.

Many nonpharmacological treatments for dementia are based on the notion that dementia care must be tailored to the unique individual. As noted by Bell and Troxel (2003), authors of *The Best Friends Approach to Dementia Care*, "If you've met one person with Alzheimer's disease, you've only met one person with Alzheimer's disease" (p. 5). What is different about the approach used in this book is that the contextual model can be used to look at individual changes in behavior over time in a systematic way. It will help you look for patterns that give clues as to what might be contributing to the presenting problem and how the situation can be changed to make things better. The contextual model can also shift the way you and your clients experience dementia symptoms so that even when they are not eliminated, they can become less distressing. The contextual model can be helpful for understanding and responding to dementia symptoms in any care setting or at any stage of disease. Thus, it is both an empirical and highly practical tool for addressing your clients' problems and concerns.

THEORETICAL BASES FOR THE CONTEXTUAL MODEL

The contextual model of dementia care integrates findings from two major areas of study: (a) *behavior analysis*—the study of how a person's cognition, affect, and behavior interact with the respective historical and current psychosocial contexts; and (b) *gerontology*—the study of age-related changes, shifting roles, and sociocultural expectations across the life span. Each of these areas makes an important contribution to a comprehensive and coherent approach to dementia care.[1]

PRINCIPLES OF BEHAVIOR ANALYSIS

Imagine a professor at an Ivy League university, famed for her brilliant lectures, who begins to stumble over words during major presentations. Her previously fluent and smooth performances in front of large audiences are now accompanied by awkward moments when speech has halted because she has lost her train of thought. How do you think the audience will respond?[2] After a while, the professor notices decreased attendance at her lectures and mentions to a colleague that students seem to avoid her. A cloud begins to settle over her professional life and her self-esteem. Now imagine a watchmaker who has worked and lived in solitude for most of his life. If he should have word-finding difficulties, do you think he would experience them in the same way as the professor? Probably not, you may say, because he is not expected to "perform" and there is no erudite audience to judge his diminished verbal performance and avoid his company. He likely will continue to enjoy his work, which is essentially unaffected by his circumscribed language deficits. These two examples illustrate how a person's life history and current circumstances mediate the social and emotional effects of the neurodegenerative disease. Behavior analysis provides the tools to help you analyze and understand these differential effects.

From a behavior analytic viewpoint, what a person says, does, or feels is functionally related to (or dependent on) the context. Reconsider the example of the professor: The loss of her audience may result in fewer invitations to speak in public, and the professor may start to avoid professional meetings that she previously enjoyed because she is worried people will notice her language difficulties. It is important to note here that it would not be sufficient to look at just a single snapshot of the professor's behavior: She still may agree

---

[1]Our integrated approach to understanding behavior in persons with dementia has been greatly influenced by the functional contextualism of Hayes et al. (Biglan & Hayes, 1996; Gifford & Hayes, 1999; Hayes, Hayes, Reese, & Sarbin, 1993) as well as by Lawton's ecological change model and its relationship to quality of life in older adults (Lawton, 1974, 1991). For more information on contextualism in the behavioral sciences, refer to http://www.contextualpsychology.org.
[2]In our daily work with individuals with dementia, we often ask ourselves how we would think, feel, and behave under similar conditions. Thus, as teachers and clinicians, the example of the professor emerged naturally, close to our heart. Fellow academics can get a glimpse of this experience in the recent compassionate and moving fictional account of a Harvard professor with early-onset Alzheimer's disease (Genova, 2009).

to give lectures here and there (behavior) even though fewer people are in attendance (context). Rather, the increased social withdrawal and loss of audience only become apparent over time and with repeated observations.

Functional analysis is the term we use to describe a hypothesis-building process of observing and trying to understand how a person's dementia symptoms may make sense in his or her particular situation. Because we are talking about human beings, rather than machines or computers, the relationship between an individual's situation (context) and their reactions to their dementia symptoms (behavior) is probabilistic, not absolute. Given a certain context, behavior is more or less likely. Stated another way, some behaviors, thoughts, or feelings will occur more frequently in some conditions and less frequently in others. Our job as health care professionals working with persons with dementia is to try to understand under what conditions various behaviors occur, so that we can help our clients and their families make changes that have a good likelihood of positively impacting their quality of life.

THE A • B • Cs OF BEHAVIOR CHANGE

So how do we begin to understand the context, or conditions, in which behaviors are more or less likely to occur? The first place to start is to look at the contingencies surrounding the behavior of interest. *Contingencies* are descriptive "if . . . then" relationships, such as, "If there are fewer attendees at each talk, then the professor will feel discouraged and the frequency of giving presentations will slowly go down." Contingencies are statements of what happens to behaviors, thoughts, or feelings over time when their context is taken into account. The contingencies of a situation can be understood by the easy-to-remember formula (A • B • C), in which A stands for antecedents or activators; B stands for the behavior of interest, which can include not only physical actions but also internal experiences such as thoughts and feelings; and C stands for consequences or what happens after B occurs.[3]

---

[3]Functional analysis of behavior dates back to B. F. Skinner's philosophy of radical behaviorism in the mid-20th century and has been widely used in clinical settings, including in work with developmentally disabled individuals. To our knowledge, the earliest application of an antecedent–behavior–consequence (ABC) model to dementia was described in Hoyer, Mishara, and Riebel (1975). It was subsequently elaborated by Hussian (1981), followed by use of functional analysis for persons with dementia by Burgio and colleagues in their work with nursing home residents (Burgio, Hardin, Sinnott, Janosky, & Hohman, 1995; Cariaga, Burgio, Flynn, & Martin, 1992) and Teri and Logsdon, who applied the three-term contingency model to the understanding and management of common mood and behavioral changes in community dwelling individuals (Teri & Logsdon, 1990). For a brief yet comprehensive treatment of the philosophy of radical behaviorism (or "contextualism") and its implications, see Chiesa (1994).

DEFINING BEHAVIORS

Building a functional analysis of the events in the lives of caregivers and care recipients (or between care recipients and us, the health care providers) is not always an easy task. The critical first step is to pick a behavior (B) to study, and then describe it in such a way that we can all agree on what we are talking about. This seemingly obvious first step is actually often the source of great difficulty when trying to get multiple family members and/or health care providers to agree on what is happening with a particular client. Several things will make this description process easier:

- Be specific. This applies not only to your description of the behavior that is the problem but also to what you want to see happen instead. The absence of behavior is not a behavior. For example, describing the problem as "Mary is not showering" is not the place to start. A better beginning would be "I want Mary to shower today, but she is refusing." Phrased this way, we know two important facts: that today is shower day and that Mary has indicated she does not want to take a shower today. This gives us a specific problem to solve and a desired timeline.
- Ask family or professional caregivers to use verbs rather than nouns or adjectives in their descriptions. It is not helpful to know that Mary is "agitated"; rather, it is more important to know what Mary was doing that led you to think she was agitated (or frightened/depressed/aggressive/frustrated/etc.). This can be especially helpful when consulting in long-term care settings, where there are frequently multiple caregivers who can have very different interpretations of and reactions to client behaviors.
- Assess the history of the specific behavior of interest. Has Mary always refused showers, or was this morning the first time? When the information is available, it is also helpful to know whether there were times before the dementia diagnosis when the behavior occurred or whether the past conditions for showering might be of relevance to the current refusal. For example, Mary's daughter might know whether Mary preferred baths to showers, whether she always took her showers in the evenings instead of mornings, or whether she always had her hair done in a salon rather than washing it at home.

CONSIDERING ACTIVATORS

Whenever something unexpected or problematic occurs, it is a natural first reaction to wonder, "Why did that happen?" The contextual model is particularly helpful here because it helps us find patterns in client behaviors that at first glimpse appear to come out of the blue. One way we look for patterns is to consider what happened before the B, or behavior of interest, occurred. *Antecedent* and *activator* are words to indicate the condition or situation that is present when behaviors, thoughts, or emotions happen. Although *antecedent* is the traditional term used in behavior analysis, we like to use the word *activator* because it makes it clearer that we are talking about a possible "why" that activates or closely relates to a behavioral problem that you want to solve. The term *activator* has a kind of energy to it; it implies that something happened and that something may be changed to make the situation better in the future.[4]

Any person, place, or thing can become an activator, and activators can be either contemporaneous with the behavior of interest or something that happened long ago. For example, when Mary refused to shower, a few activators you might want to consider include the particular staff person who came to help her, the way that staff person worded the shower request, or the fact that Mary had recently gotten back from breakfast and was tired. Common to all activator situations is that they provide the context in which a certain behavior is more (or less) likely to occur. Your question is: What happens to Mary's behavior when showering conditions are changed, when a different staff person invites her to shower or asks her with a different tone of voice or at a different time of day? When searching for potential activators, you might also consider the manner in which Mary refused to shower. For example, if she said, "I will take my next shower in the spring," you might wonder whether a warm towel and bathrobe, or a warmer room or water temperature would make her more likely to agree to shower today. Note, the activator context is not a "trigger" in the sense that when A happens, B will always follow. If we change the staff person or room temperature, Mary might still refuse showers but perhaps not as frequently as before. Human beings are not machines who respond the same way each time they experience similar circumstances. That is because there are sometimes more subtle, implicit, or historical factors embedded in a situation that also influence what we choose and how we act.

---

[4]Actually, neither the term *activator* nor its traditional alternative *antecedent* is ideal in this context. Both terms are problematic to the extent that they imply we should be looking for a simple push–pull mechanism that "triggers" the problem behavior in contiguous time. A preferable A term might be *actifying situation*, which could refer to either past or present events that energize or strengthen the probability of the behavior occurring. However, that would be an awkward substitution, so we will use *activator*, with the admonition to the reader to remember that discrete stimuli occurring immediately prior to the behavior are not exclusively what we mean and that people who only look for these will be disappointed.

UNDERSTANDING CONSEQUENCES

The third element to the A • B • C contingency description is what happens after a behavior occurs. *Consequences* are events that follow the behavior, thoughts, or feelings of interest. Once behaviors occur, they are either maintained and supported or discouraged and diminished by their consequences. Behavior analysts use the terms *reinforcement* and *punishment* to distinguish how consequences alter the frequency, magnitude, intensity, or other quality of a person's behavior over time.

Increasing Behaviors: Reinforcement

A *positive reinforcing event* is a consequence that increases the likelihood that a behavior will occur again or continue. The care recipient who is given chocolate ice cream when she asks for dessert is likely to ask for dessert again tomorrow. However, it is important to note that positive reinforcement is not the same thing as an intentional "reward." There are two reasons for this. First, we do not know whether an event will function as a reinforcer until we have observed its effect on behavior over time. Reinforcement is highly personal and idiosyncratic. The care recipient's requests for dessert may slowly subside if she is always given canned peaches instead of chocolate ice cream (even though the less preferred peaches may be a more healthy eating choice). Whether a person has a dementia diagnosis or not, preferences count. In the care of people with dementia, participation in pleasant activities is often recommended. However, not just any activity will do. Rather, we need to find activities that reinforce (i.e., maintain and support) participation. Truly reinforcing events are usually meaningful to the person and relevant to his or her history. They may not always be what we would consider "rewarding"; for example, a person who used to work as a nurse may enjoy making beds more than she enjoys playing bingo. Reinforcements are also often intrinsic to our interactions, as opposed to rewards that are contrived. Talking, telling stories, and sharing experiences, for example, are naturally reinforcing for most people. We do not need gold stars on our foreheads or a pat on the back every time we see our best friend to increase the likelihood we will want to see him or her tomorrow.

Many behaviors of individuals with dementia can also be negatively reinforced. This term is easily confused with punishment. Instead, *negative reinforcement* means that a person will be more likely to engage in a behavior if that behavior reliably helps to avoid or escape from an unwanted situation. In practice, the behavior of individuals with dementia is often negatively rather than positively reinforced. A common example is the client who becomes impatient and insists on leaving when her neurologist tries to administer a mental status exam at her annual visit. In other cases, individuals with dementia come to use question-terminating platitudes or truisms to avoid or escape from such demand situations. Using the A • B • Cs, consider the following exchange between a neurologist and her client:

Neurologist: How old are you? [A]

Client: One doesn't ask a lady for her age. [B]

Consequence [C]: Neurologist drops demand for information and moves on to the next question.

Neurologist: What is this? [She points to her watch; A]

Client: I do not like putting names on things. [B]

Consequence [C]: Neurologist moves on to the next question.

Neurologist: What season is it? [A]

Client: I think it is spring, but we can agree to disagree. [B]

Consequence [C]: Neurologist moves on to the next question.

We can speculate that individuals who consistently respond to questions in this fashion live in a social environment that has respected their authority and treated such utterances as acceptable answers. From the contextual model, the person with dementia is not making an intentional attempt at a clever deception. Instead, he or she likely has a history of using graceful social maneuvers to escape from uncomfortable situations. In the example, the neurologist stopped asking the client questions to which she did not know the answers. Her gentle evasion strategy was reinforced, and the client is likely to use it again.

Decreasing Behaviors: Punishment

The term *punishment* is scary to many people because in common parlance it usually means retribution or retaliation. In functional analysis, however, punishment simply means that a consequence decreases the likelihood that a behavior will occur again. The following example will illustrate how the A • B • Cs can be used to better understand the situation.

A caregiver comes to your office and is distressed because her severely impaired spouse is "unwilling" to talk to her. You observe the care recipient when he is with his wife and also when he is alone with you or with other members of your staff. You notice that he easily and charmingly engages in banter with any of your staff members and laughs with them (activator situation 1) but that he almost never talks in the presence of his wife (activator situation 2). When you examine the difference between the staff's and the caregiver's stances, you find that your staff members—aware of the severity of the person's dementia—do not correct the person's utterances, do not fill in for him, and do not hold his verbal performance to any "truth criterion." As trained by you, they go with the flow of taking turns, nodding, and laughing, making the conversation easy and relatively content free. In other words, they try to be "on the same page" as the person with dementia, to carefully read nonverbal cues of comfort and discomfort, and to respond to his remarks with generally pleasant conversational and "small-talk" topics (consequence 1). The result is the person with dementia engages in conversation (behavior 1). The caregiver, in contrast, tries to orient her husband to reality, corrects his mistakes, and fills in words when he takes too long to answer your questions (consequence 2). Her sentences are long and complex, and she seems visibly upset when her husband is "uncooperative." The caregiver's attempts to recover the conversations she once had with her husband thus may have inadvertently punished his verbal responsiveness; that is, the frequency of utterances in his wife's presence have decreased over time (behavior 2).

Notice that the caregiver in our example is well intentioned: She is not trying to "punish" her husband, in the everyday sense of the term, but only trying to maintain her previous relationship with him. Yet, functionally, her husband's behavior decreases in rate, and a punishment contingency is in effect. Recent research in our universities (University of Washington, University of Nevada–Reno) has shown that family caregivers can be coached to eliminate these punishing interactional patterns and to effectively engage their loved ones yet again (Gentry & Fisher, 2007). It is also important to note that although in this case, the wife's correction and filling in appears to be functioning as a punisher for your client (i.e., it decreases his verbal responsiveness), another individual with dementia might perceive his spouse's similar efforts as supportive and helpful. What functions as reinforcement or punishment (i.e., what increases or decreases the behavior of interest) for one person does not automatically have similar functions for another person.

Negative punishment is a consequence that decreases behavior by decreasing access to reinforcing events. This kind of contingency is familiar to every parent and sports fan under the names "time-out" and "penalty." To illustrate inadvertent negative punishment contingencies inherent in many caregiver–care recipient interactions, we often tell the ancient parable of the man who found a butterfly working hard to exit a cocoon. Reluctant to merely observe a presumably struggling creature and eager to help, the man pried a hole into the cocoon. Little did he know that the premature release prohibited the pumping of fluids into the butterfly's wings, a prerequisite for flying. Observing a care recipient struggle with a task, many well-intentioned caregivers tend to take the task away: "Here, let *me* do this." The care recipient, as a consequence, is denied the opportunity to engage in any challenging activity, which may mean loss of all opportunities to feel successful and competent. Caregivers often are particularly perplexed by the fine line between being helpful and being controlling or patronizing. The contextual model provides the tools for individual analyses as to what strategies work for which persons in a variety of situations.

Fading Consequences: Extinction

In general, consequences only work best to increase or decrease behaviors as long as they are presented following the behavior of interest. When punishment contingencies are discontinued, the behavior previously affected can increase to former levels. If the caregiver in our previous example learns to stop inadvertently punishing her husband's speaking by correcting him, contextual theory would predict that his conversations with his wife would increase.

Similarly, when reinforcement contingencies involving a valued or meaningful activity are withdrawn or discontinued, a person's engagement in that particular activity will slowly decrease. From the perspective of the contextual model, this latter situation is highly significant. Dementia profoundly restricts our clients' opportunities for positive reinforcement. Just think of the retiree who spent most of her day playing golf and who is now confined to the house because of way-finding difficulties, or the amateur restorer of antique clocks who cannot set the pendulum, let alone open the case, and may now be looking at his clocks with helpless despair because they are all telling different time. A significant part of providing behavioral health care within the contextual model consists of discovering and implementing novel reinforcing events that can function to activate the person and improve his or her mood.

Behavior Shaped by Contingencies

Activators and consequences are important shapers of our behavior throughout the life span. For example, many of our social skills are not explicitly taught but are acquired by experience and watching other people. Based on activators and consequences inherent in the context, we develop "gut feelings" or automatic reactions to situations which we may find difficult to describe and often equally difficult to change. Behavior analysts say these feelings and reactions are *contingency-shaped*; that is, they are patterns of behavior that have never been explicitly instructed. Rather, they have emerged over a lifetime with repeated exposure to similar combinations of activators and consequences. It is important for dementia care providers to know that contingency-shaped social patterns tend to persist and that most individuals with significant cognitive impairment retain their ability to respond differentially to social cues even when the ability to comprehend language or express ideas has been severely compromised (Hubbard, Cook, Tester, & Downs, 2002). Thus, a physician's exclusive attention to the caregiver during an intake interview may be upsetting to even a severely impaired care recipient, who may not verbally understand what is being discussed but retains the social expectation that he should be able to speak for himself in the doctor's office. Retained contingency-shaped behaviors, such as excellent social skills, often prompt caregivers to overestimate a person's cognitive abilities and to become irritated when the care recipient is unable to perform seemingly simple tasks.

Routines may also establish activators and consequences in a noninstructed, contingency-shaped fashion. Being a "creature of habit" translates into a daily life filled with activator cues setting the occasion for one activity following the next. As we all know, well-established routines can generate the feeling of being "on autopilot." In these seemingly effortlessly executed chain performances, the consequences of one completed step become the activator for the next step, as when we take a shower and follow a predictable sequence of taking off our clothes, turning on the water, stepping into the shower, washing our body and hair, rinsing off the soap, turning off the water, stepping out, and toweling dry.

As dementia progresses, every step along common chained routines becomes a potential place to stumble and often requires supplemental prompting or modeling. "What do I do next?" is a question frequently posed by individuals with dementia in many different forms and indicates that the influence of formerly well-established A • B • (C = A) • B • (C = A) chains in a person's life is breaking down. In our bathing example, we skipped many steps actually necessary for a complete task analysis of taking a shower, such as entering the bathroom, making sure a towel for drying off is nearby, testing the combination of hot and cold water to get the perfect temperature, finding the soap and shampoo and using each appropriately, and bridging the duration of turning on the water and stepping into the shower without getting distracted by other, more immediate, events. Each step is another place for the person with dementia to get "derailed" and wind up wandering off distracted or simply stopping the sequence altogether.

GERONTOLOGICAL THEORY AND PERSON–ENVIRONMENT FIT

Although some of our behavior may be contingency-shaped, many influential activator and consequent conditions are also verbal. Rules, concepts, inferences, judgments, values, reasons, explanations, rationales, or worldviews are all verbal belief systems or habits that affect our behavior in various ways. We are taught as we grow up in schools, families, or communities that our actions and life events or circumstances are likely to (or should) take a certain form, and we are puzzled, saddened, confused, or angered when they do not happen as we expect. We pay special attention to the influence of these learned, verbal contingencies throughout the book, because they often generate real dilemmas for people with dementia and their caregivers.

For example, many persons with dementia resist assistance with personal care such as bathing or toileting because we are all taught early in life to value privacy and autonomy. Many caregivers are reluctant to place family members in nursing homes long after care at home has become overwhelming because of promises made to the loved one years ago or because a caregiver has negative stereotypes about the kind of care you get "in those places" (that the caregiver may have never visited). Psychosocial and historical familial, religious, and cultural expectations create a set of verbal "rules" that affect the relative importance that each of us places on our autonomy, physical and cognitive health, role identities, work and recreational habits, and social support networks. *Gerontological theory*[5] talks about the importance of a good person–environment fit for maintenance of quality of life. Verbal contingencies can either make it more difficult for individuals with dementia and their caregivers to find the best fit for their dementia care needs or, conversely, can lead to great inner strength and flexibility. Thus, consideration of the broader psychosocial history and context is as important as events in the environment if we wish to understand the development and possible solutions for dementia-related behavior changes.

CONDUCTING A FUNCTIONAL ANALYSIS

Table 2.1 provides an overview of how the A • B • Cs are considered in practical application. Taken together, these steps are called a *functional analysis* of behavior. When events are considered in this way, we quickly begin to see that it is possible for two behaviors to appear quite different from one another and yet produce the same outcome. As an example, Rosita, who has mild dementia, still lives alone in her home. Her daughter, Grace, who stops by every day, notices one day that Rosita's storm door is broken. Wanting to help her mother, Grace takes Rosita to a large, noisy home improvement center. Standing in a long aisle lined with storm doors, Grace and Rosita look up and down at door after door. When Grace asks Rosita, "So, Mom, which storm door would you like?" Rosita suddenly exclaims, "Stop bossing me around!" An argument ensues, and Grace takes Rosita home. The storm

---

[5]Persons interested in knowing more about gerontological theory are referred to Lawton (1974, 1991).

TABLE 2.1
Overview of Steps in the ABCs

Activators	Behaviors	Consequences
Examine historical and proximal activators: When, where, around whom, how often does the behavior occur?	*Specify behavior of interest:* What exactly is the client doing that you would like to see change?	*Consider immediate consequences:* How do people respond? Over time, has the behavior been increasing or decreasing in frequency? What does the behavior accomplish?
Rosita is at the store with Grace who wants her to select a storm door. The store is busy and noisy. This is the first time this has happened.	Rosita yells at her daughter to stop bossing her around.	Grace gets angry and takes Rosita home. Grace does not take her mother back to the store to get a new door.
Consider the broader psychosocial context: How has dementia changed the client's roles, activities, and access to family and friends? How do the client's family and friends perceive cognitive impairment?	*Gather a behavioral history:* Is this a new behavior, or has it happened before? Does it fit into a long-standing pattern? Is it a sudden onset or gradual change?	*Conduct a general reinforcer assessment:* Does the client have things in her or his life that bring joy or give life meaning?

door remains broken. These events are summarized in bold text in the second row of Table 2.1.

Rosita's yelling at her daughter in the hardware store was negatively reinforced when it led to her daughter taking her home and away from the overwhelming array of storm doors. Negative reinforcement principles would thus predict that in the future, Rosita would be more likely to yell when she is in a situation where she feels anxious or trapped. However, it is useful to note that any behavior that would have allowed Rosita to escape from the overwhelming demand of choosing a storm door for her home could be classified into the same functional class as her yelling at her daughter. Rosita could have said, "Take me home" or "Why don't we get something to eat? I think my blood sugar is dropping" or "I don't like any of these doors." She could have started crying, she could have complained about the price of home repair, or she could have accused family members of financial exploitation. Although each of these reactions topographically appears different, they would belong in the same functional class if they brought about a similar result, namely, Grace taking her mother home. Thus, when using the A • B • Cs to help understand behaviors in persons with dementia, it is important to ask the caregiver what the behavior accomplished. The most effective interventions modify entire functional classes rather than single, isolated instances of behavior and affect. In other words, we do not just want to help Rosita get some new screen doors. We want her daughter to understand that making complex decisions in highly stimulating situations is hard for Rosita now, and a different approach needs to be taken.

If you were working with Rosita and Grace, you would want to know a little bit about Rosita's broader psychosocial context and the history of her relationship with Grace before the store episode. Has Rosita always relied on her daughter to help with home repairs, or is this a recent change? Did Rosita and Grace have a good relationship in the past, or did they often argue? Is Rosita still involved with her friends and valued activities, or has she become increasingly isolated at home? Those kinds of questions are found in the second row of Table 2.1. Although we are not elaborating on them now for our screen door example with Rosita and Grace, we will see in the clinical cases that follow in later chapters how such background information is an important part of A • B • C functional analyses and invaluable in developing effective treatment plans with our clients.

TAKING THE CONTEXTUAL MODEL INTO THE REAL WORLD

The remainder of this book is organized in such a way as to show readers how to apply the contextual model with multiple clients and a range of presenting problems. We encourage you throughout to notice the focus on patterns: From the contextual model of dementia, behaviors generally do not come out of the blue but can be understood in terms of the person's history, his or her psychosocial and sociocultural contexts, and his or her immediate environment and situation, as well as in terms of the progressive neurodegenerative changes predicted by the disorder. In the following chapters, we systematically show you how to consider these various contexts at every stage of dementia care, including diagnostic assessments, referrals, treatment, and long-term care planning. The contextual model will enable you to identify multiple strategies for intervention, suggest expert solutions, and examine their outcomes.

The contextual model of dementia care requires practitioners to juggle a lot of balls concurrently, and the complexity and multitude of issues to consider can be challenging. To help you, we have developed a simple approach, a set of clinical guidelines from which you practice your contextual skills. These guidelines are in the form of the acronym *DANCE*. In the next chapter, we examine the DANCE and its application as you are introduced to your first case.

II

THE DEMENTIA DANCE
FOR CLINICIANS

3

BUILD COLLABORATIVE
RELATIONSHIPS

The foundation of good dementia care can be compared to a three-legged stool: Every leg is important for keeping things in balance. In Chapter 1, we discussed the importance of the first leg: the dementia diagnosis. Part of the diagnostic process is examining the client's unique pattern of cognitive and behavioral symptoms. Every brain disease is different. Every person living with dementia experiences and responds to it differently. That is what makes the second leg of the stool—the contextual model of dementia care presented in Chapter 2—so useful. A knowledge of activators and consequences, about what reinforces (increases) behavior and what punishes (decreases) behavior, is invaluable for trying to make sense of the individual differences and seeming unpredictability exhibited by persons with dementia. The contextual model is also at the heart of effective treatment. Functional analysis shows us that behaviors associated with dementia occur in a context that includes the here and now (i.e., "What just happened and what did you do about it?") and also the client's unique personal history (i.e., "How is this similar to or different from how he reacted in the past?"). The more you can come to understand the context, the "big picture" of a person's life, the better positioned you will be to help both care recipients and caregivers.

The third leg of the stool is the relationship you build with your clients and the attitude or posture you assume toward their disease and symptoms. Unlike the care of persons with chronic diseases such as hypertension or diabetes, which can be managed with medications or healthier patterns of eating or exercising, treatment of persons with cognitive decline almost always involves work at the interpersonal level. Effective dementia care creates a psychosocial environment that fosters meaningful activity and prevents social withdrawal. It institutes reinforcement (e.g., increases in pleasurable activity and interpersonal connection) and tries to eliminate punishment contingencies (e.g., decreases in engagement) in the client's life by changing his or her social environment. To that end, it promotes acceptance and understanding of the incurable aspects of the dementing illness, while at the same time generating hope for improved quality of life. When you are able to relate to your clients with empathy, respect, flexibility, and genuine regard, you can make a difference in their lives.

INTEGRATING DIAGNOSIS, CONTEXT, AND RELATIONSHIP: THE DEMENTIA DANCE

In 2006, one of us (Sue) published a book for family caregivers, *When a Family Member Has Dementia: Steps to Becoming a Resilient Caregiver* (McCurry, 2006). An early chapter of the book told the story of a woman with advanced dementia who refused to bathe and her spouse who solved the problem by putting on music and dancing her into the shower. In this story, the caregiver gave up trying to convince his wife that her hygiene was slipping. Instead, he took advantage of his intimate knowledge of his wife's preferences and pleasures to find a spontaneous solution to his dilemma. The dance came to symbolize creative problem solving as well as the sophistication and flexibility necessary to think of noncoercive and affable solutions that maintain the trusting relationship between caregiver and care recipient. To enable other family caregivers to engage in similarly gracious behavior, Sue proposed a simple set of core strategies based on the metaphor of dancing and the acronym DANCE. This acronym and its components have since proved useful not only in our work with family caregivers but also with health care colleagues and our trainees. With these fellow professionals, we often found ourselves playing with and slightly modifying the original acronym to make it a useful clinical guide. This modified version is what we want to share with you:

- D: Discuss concerns respectfully.
- A: Ameliorate excess disability.
- N: Nurture the dyad.
- C: Create contextual solutions.
- E: Enjoy the journey.

Discuss Concerns Respectfully

For family caregivers, the admonition we used was, "Don't argue!" Argument, logic, and verbal persuasion all become increasingly ineffective with persons with dementia as they lose their ability to remember what you are talking about or follow the reasonable explanation you are trying so carefully to make. It is not helpful to insist that your wife has not bathed in a week when she is certain she took a shower just this morning. Shouting at your husband for digging up the prize roses will not prevent him from trying to help in the garden tomorrow, particularly if keeping up the yard was his responsibility for decades. Family members who live with someone with progressive dementia must learn new ways to listen to and talk with the care recipient, ways that will help persons with dementia maintain both their dignity and a safe and healthy lifestyle. Families will come to you, the health care professional, to teach them how to do this and to model effective communication skills. They will also come to you in the hope that you will know just the right words to say and have the right tone of voice or authority to deliver bad news in such a way that will make the difficult transition easy for everyone. What family members want is for the therapist to say, "Mr. Jones, you need to give up driving," "Mrs. Smith, it is time to move out of your home of 55 years and into assisted living," and for Mr. Jones and Mrs. Smith to listen, nod thoughtfully, and say, "Oh, yes, when you put it that way, of course I can see that is what must be done."

Unfortunately, even the most skilled professionals are not wonder workers with communication tricks up their sleeves. What we are asking of individuals with dementia and their families is hard. Functional analyses and the contextual model of care can suggest solutions for many of the behavioral and emotional problems associated with cognitive decline, but their implementation requires care recipients to accept assistance or changes in routines, and caregivers to alter their style of interaction with the care recipient. This takes time and dialogue, and the best behavioral health care plans will fail if we have not understood the big picture. One of our clients took care of his spouse who was unable to communicate or initiate actions because of advanced dementia. The caregiver's own disability prevented him from physically prompting and assisting his wife with transfers from a lying to a sitting or standing position. We suggested the purchase of a hospital bed to facilitate the transfer. The caregiver agreed to the suggestion but never followed through with the purchase. Only months later, after the family caregiver had hired outside help to aid his wife's transfers, did we find out that the caregiver's wish to continue holding his wife at night had been the barrier to moving to separate beds. Care recipients and caregivers both need to feel that their unique situation is understood, and if that does not happen, they will not take our recommendations to heart.

Ameliorate Excess Disability

Before caregivers can accept that a family member has a dementia diagnosis, accept the gamut of behavioral changes and limitations that will follow, and accept their own emotional roller coaster reactions, they have to feel that everything possible to reverse the situation has been tried. This is where you, the health care professional, come in. Before starting down the road of contextual problem solving, you have to help rule out treatable factors that might be causing or worsening the person with dementia's situation and make sure that appropriate treatments are implemented, either by you or a referral colleague.

Excess disability is a term used to describe the circumstance in which someone with dementia is doing worse than predicted by the diagnosed neurodegenerative disease because of the added burden of physical or psychiatric disease. If we have a bad day or "feel not up to snuff," our performance may deteriorate. For individuals with dementia, such deterioration can be drastic in the face of unmanaged disease, undetected sensory loss, depression, anxiety, or medication side effects. As pointed out previously, early communicative deficits in dementia may produce an inability to clearly describe one's own physiological or psychological condition. People who are still able to comment on local politics may not be able to point to localized pain, such as from urinary tract infections, or to describe stomach upset or constipation. Someone else who always been able to change his hearing aid batteries without difficulty may suddenly fail to do so and experience acute hearing loss that presents similarly to delirium and highly unusual confusion. Frustration over being unable to think clearly, depression about anticipated lifestyle changes or losses, and worry about future problems such as having to move into residential care or becoming a burden to family can all worsen cognitive symptoms. Before conducting a functional analysis, it is necessary to systematically rule out excess disability related to comorbidities, anxiety, depression, or sensory loss.

Similarly, medications play an important role as potential sources of excess disability in dementia care. Many cognitively impaired individuals are taking at least one medication prescribed to slow cognitive decline or to stabilize mood or behavior. Frequently, side effects of these medications outweigh their intended and anticipated cognitive, emotional, or behavioral benefits. Even medications for chronic diseases that have been well-tolerated for years may begin to adversely affect a person's condition because of changes in weight or metabolic status. To make matters more precarious, nowadays polymedicine is a part of aging: A 2002 survey found that almost all ambulatory, noninstitutionalized men and women over 65 years of age took at least one medication, more than half took five or more, and 12% took 10 or more (Kaufman, Kelly, Rosenberg, Anderson, & Mitchell, 2002). The number of medications taken is a predictor of adverse events, and the majority of individuals with dementia take more than one medication. Although the ideal for good medical care is that all older adults, including persons with dementia, have one primary care "gatekeeper" who monitors all medication prescriptions and referrals to health care specialists, in practice that does not always turn out to be the case. Thus, it sometimes will fall to you to review with caregivers who is treating the care recipient, what medications have been prescribed and what medications are actually being taken, including those that are purchased over the counter; from naturopaths, the Internet, or health food stores; or even borrowed from family and friends.

Nurture the Dyad

Persons with dementia and their caregivers come to you, the health care professional, because they want and need help. This help comes in many forms. Your health care expertise is an essential part of making the dementia diagnosis, evaluating the care recipient's cognitive and functional status, identifying and treating any comorbid physical or psychiatric conditions that worsen the situation, and problem solving for solutions to thorny behavioral challenges. However, you also can provide an invaluable service by helping both the caregiver and care recipient find self-worth, satisfaction, and even joy as they learn to live with a dementia diagnosis and its progression.

Persons with dementia experience many blows to their personal identity when they get the diagnosis. Family and friends often treat them differently, or at least the care recipient perceives that to be the case. There are fewer visitors and invitations to social events; it is easier to quit the weekly bridge game than to be "invited" to play at a less competitive table. Lapses in memory, forgotten names, and minor word-finding slips are all a daily reminder that "I am losing my mind." Many activities that have been sources of pleasure are set aside: traveling, hunting, woodworking, sewing, solitary walks after dark. Both care recipients and caregivers just want things to be "normal," but the new normal includes changing roles that can be hard to accept. Adult children take over the parent's finances. One spouse takes over all the driving, another learns how to cook and do laundry. For care recipients, each change is a loss. For caregivers, in addition to loss, each change brings a new responsibility. You, the health care professional, may be the only person the dyad knows who can help both the caregiver and care recipient look beyond the many hard and scary changes that dementia brings and to find continued life purpose and meaning.

As persons with dementia and their family members scramble to make sense of their new reality, you might find them at one or another emotional or behavioral extreme: stating that all is lost because of the disease or engaging in wishful thinking about a cure, adamantly refusing help or desperately

seeking it, offering assistance to the care recipient or categorically withdrawing it on encountering resistance. Concurrent emotions run the gamut from
shame, anger, and fear to love and pity. We, as dementia care providers, teach
and model the coexistence of acceptance and hope as well as safety and self-
determination. These are not mutually exclusive constructs, although for many
clients—and providers—they may appear so initially. Caregivers often do not
only ask "What should I do" but also "How should I feel?" Nurturing the dyad
includes validating such confusing emotions and helping caregivers and care
recipients alike find ways to continue to enjoy much that is still beautiful and
pleasant in the world.

Create Contextual Solutions

As we described earlier, good dementia care acknowledges the idiosyncratic nature of neurodegenerative diseases. A number of evidence-based treatments for behavioral disturbances in dementia have been developed, and
we help you become aware of these in this book. However, implicit in all such
dementia care interventions is the need to individualize treatment to suit the
particular situation. This requires both closely examining current circumstances and also taking a detailed history to detect relevant activators and
consequences. One care recipient, for example, suddenly refused to get into
the passenger side of the car. He would gladly sit in the back seat or enter a
bus, but his spouse was not able to prompt him to ride in the front passenger
seat. The caregiver was at a loss to understand this change until she recalled
that the care recipient grew up in Australia and spent his young adult years
there—driving on the left. Once the caregiver realized that asking her spouse
to enter the passenger side of the car was equivalent to asking him to drive,
she abandoned her attempts to coax him into the passenger seat. Thus, effective problem solving often requires putting aside our own ideas about "what
is right" so we can figure out "what will work" in the situation. Contextual
problem solving is not only helpful for common affective and behavioral
changes in dementia but also for trying to find meaningful areas of engagement and activity to prevent depression and social withdrawal and for examining potential barriers to change on the caregiver's side.

There is an art to creating contextual solutions. Most important, we
must be sensitive to caregiver and care recipient personal preferences and
values and respect their solution choices. For example, when dementia is
progressive and reasoning skills decline, there usually comes a time when
providing logical facts (reality orientation) is not consistently helpful. The
caregiver may tell a person who insists on "going home" while in his own
house, "You *are* at home. Don't you remember, we bought this house and
moved in 40 years ago?" However, the care recipient may perceive this

response as argumentative. He may become defensive and feel rejected instead of reassured. In considering alternative responses with the caregiver, it is important to talk through their implications in a collaborative way. What guidelines can the caregiver use to decide that a logical explanation may not be best? How can family members know when it is time to switch from providing cues and corrective reminders to using compassionate misinformation ("We'll be going home in a little while") or benign deceptions (e.g., getting into the car and driving around the block then pulling up into the driveway and announcing "We're home now")? How do you address caregivers' concerns that this is "lying" or "tricking" a loved one? When would it be more appropriate to enter the care recipient's experiential realm and validate his or her feelings by saying, "Yes, I imagine nothing looks familiar to you, and you're longing for a safe place"? Alternatively, how do you and the family decide that a person cannot live alone in his or her home, and it is time to pursue assisted living or memory care? How will you secure the care recipient's collaboration? Contextual problem solving will be most effective when we learn to listen to what caregivers and care recipients are saying they need and want and then help them achieve these goals rather than dictating our own best professional opinions.

Enjoy Sharing the Journey

When you become part of a caregiving journey, you have the privilege to witness and participate in genuine human connections. As language skills diminish, many of the negative aspects of being able to reason and argue also fall by the wayside. Importantly, declining cognitive functioning may mean that relationships that were clouded by a person's rules, reasoning, and arguments can actually improve; parents who were highly critical of their children's same-sex partners may start enjoying their time with them, spouses who used to be highly bound to the "shoulds" and "oughts" of traditional divisions of labor may come to value the opportunity to develop unfamiliar skills. Opportunities for new experiences also sometimes emerge. One of our clients tells the "olive story": Her husband had always avoided olives because he said he was allergic to them. He would go to Mexican restaurants and order dishes without olives. If even one olive appeared on his plate for decorative purposes, he would leave the restaurant, claiming he could not trust the chef. On developing Lewy body dementia and being placed in a specialized Alzheimer's care unit, a staff member noticed that the husband was eating another resident's nachos and immediately called the caregiver. Together, they monitored his reaction, but there was no adverse physical effect. Rather, the husband seemed to greatly enjoy this new cuisine. Ever after, he picked out olives from dishes and expressed much pleasure in eating them.

When self-stated rules of conduct break down, there is opportunity to reunite families, to improve relationships, and to open up new pleasurable experiences, such as eating olives. Many caregivers describe having a "true" connection with their loved one, sharing laughter and pleasant activities as well as experiencing intense heart-to-heart encounters they never had before. The various steps of the DANCE create a space in which our modern emphasis on rationality and memory as prerequisites to dignity and respect and to quality of life can be abandoned. It then becomes possible to appreciate and cherish the person with dementia for who they are, who they have been, and, yes, even who they are becoming. At the same time, dementia care can be at times difficult and exhausting. There are some caregivers and care recipients who challenge our ability to see the good in our shared journey. In these cases, you will see that the same DANCE steps can be helpful in building nonjudgmental working relationships from which you can provide quality care.

APPLYING THE DEMENTIA DANCE: A CASE EXAMPLE

The DANCE acronym offers an easy-to-remember road map for assessment and treatment, for building relationships that are flexible, respectful, and applicable to a diverse range of cognitively impaired clients and situations. It emphasizes an unhurried posture from which to approach a caring relationship with cognitively impaired individuals and their family members over the entire course of disease progression. Good dementia care is like a kind of dance, a give and take, a balance between offering expert solutions and establishing close collaborative relationships that consider clients' preferences and concerns.

Throughout this book, we use several cases to illustrate how expert knowledge of dementia and the contextual model of care actually play out in the DANCE, both for the person with dementia and for you, the health care provider, at each point in time. The cases we have chosen reflect a range of typical situations that a health care provider is likely to encounter. You will see how to ask the right questions, when to consult with other professionals and agencies, and how to develop strategies for reducing affective and behavioral changes and enhancing client quality of life. We show how clients can be involved in respectful decision making throughout the continuum of care. Finally, with each case we demonstrate how caregivers' and the health care practitioners' own histories and socioenvironmental contexts need to be considered in good dementia care. Let us take a look at the first case and its implications for effective dementia care, given what you have learned so far.

CASE 1. MRS. SMITH: HELPING BLENDED
FAMILIES ADJUST TO NEW ROLES

Mrs. Smith is an 80-year-old woman who lives with her daughter, Mary, and Mary's family in Mrs. Smith's home. Mrs. Smith is a retired nurse's aide who is particular about her personal appearance. She recently moved out of a board and care facility where she had resided for the past 6 months because her own home did not sell and she could no longer afford to pay the monthly facility rent. There had also been problems in the board and care residence because Mrs. Smith was very independent and disliked being told what to do. In the facility, she complained about community meals and "set the kitchen on fire" trying to fix her own breakfast. She insisted on continuing to drive until she caused an accident. She refused any assistance with personal care. When reminded that it was time to take her medication or go to a doctor's appointment, Mrs. Smith would become angry and hit, shove, scratch, or push whoever was within arm's reach. She wandered away from the home on several occasions. Her behavioral challenges and resistance to care led to multiple psychiatric hospitalization stays. Mary, her husband, and their teenaged son have now moved in with Mrs. Smith to provide much-needed 24-hr supervision, but Mrs. Smith frequently accuses them of stealing her money, trying to poison her, and planning to lock her up in an institution. A review of Mrs. Smith's medical records shows a recent Mini-Mental State Examination (MMSE; Folstein, Folstein, & McHugh, 1975) score of 11/30.[1] Mary is seeking an appointment with you to discuss whether Mrs. Smith can remain at home or needs to be permanently placed in a long-term care community.

This is a fairly typical example of the kind of information that you would be given before a first visit with a new dementia client and caregiving family. Following DANCE principles and the knowledge of what issues are important regarding the dementia diagnosis and the context in which problems

---

[1]The MMSE (Folstein et al., 1975) is the most widely used cognitive screening test in the world (Mossello & Boncinelli, 2006). Total possible scores range from 0 to 30, with higher scores indicating less cognitive impairment. A score of less than 24 was recommended in the original source article as indicative of dementia for persons with at least 8 years of education, but this detection threshold is highly sensitive to age, level of education, and literacy (Mitchell, 2009; Tombaugh & McIntyre, 1992). In particular, the MMSE often underestimates cognitive impairment in persons with high premorbid intelligence and educational level or in those with early stage disease.

For reviews describing other cognitive, mood, behavior, and functional assessment screening tools for persons with dementia, and discussion of issues related to reliability, validity, and clinical use beyond the scope of this book, see Appendix A as well as American Geriatrics Society and American Association of Geriatric Psychiatry (2003b); Burns, Lawlor, and Craig (2002); Lezak (1995); Perrault, Oremus, Demers, Vida, and Wolfson (2000); Sikkes, de Lange-de Klerk, Pijnenburg, Scheltens, and Uitdehaag (2009); Spreen and Strauss (1998); Strober and Arnett (2009); and Teri and Logsdon (1995).

have developed, what questions might you want to explore when you meet with Mrs. Smith and her daughter? The following are some suggestions:

- D: Discuss concerns respectfully. From what you have been told, it seems fairly clear that Mrs. Smith does suffer from dementia. However, is there any information from her psychiatric hospitalizations regarding what kind of dementia she has? Did she see a neurologist? Was any cognitive testing done to evaluate her dementia severity? Is there a primary doctor for whom you will want permission to obtain medical records? How does Mrs. Smith see her situation? How will you build rapport and evaluate her cognitive strengths and weaknesses, given her fear that she is going to be institutionalized? Does Mary really want to figure out how to keep Mrs. Smith at home, or is she at her wits' end and looking to you for information about an exit plan? What is the best way to gather information from both Mrs. Smith and her daughter, given their differences in opinion about what she needs?

- A: Ameliorate excess disability. Has Mrs. Smith's cognitive decline been slowly progressive, or was there a rapid onset in the board and care home? How do the psychiatric institutionalizations relate to Mrs. Smith's decline? Does she have any known medical conditions that could be worsening her situation? Have medical tests been conducted to rule out treatable, reversible causes of dementia? Is her suspicion about her family's intentions a lifelong tendency given family relationship patterns or a history of psychiatric problems, or is it a recent development since her multiple hospitalizations (or since she lost her hearing aids)? What psychotropic medications has she been prescribed? Could they be causing side effects or interacting with other medication?

- N: Nurture the dyad. Are there particular people or situations around which Mrs. Smith does best? What brings her pleasure, relieves her anxiety, or just generally makes her easier or more enjoyable to be around? How long has Mary been a primary caregiver for her mom? How is she managing being "sandwiched" between caring for Mrs. Smith and managing the usual household responsibilities of wife and mother? How much are Mrs. Smith and her family able to get away from one another to do things they enjoy? What is the family's economic situation; might they need referrals to social services for assistance?

- C: Create contextual solutions. Mary described a number of situations in which her mother has had difficulty (see Table 3.1).

TABLE 3.1
Initiating Use of the ABCs With Mrs. Smith

Activators	Behaviors	Consequences
	Refusing to accept help with personal care	
	Unsafe self-directed behaviors (driving, cooking)	
	Verbal (accusing) and physical (hitting, shoving, scratching, pushing) behavior, interpreted as "aggressive" by the caregiver	
	Wandering	

As you gather more information about the A • B • Cs of these events, can any pattern—any common functional class of behaviors—be found? When, where, around whom, and how often do these problems occur? Are there details about Mrs. Smith's past life that would give you insight into her actions? What do her problematic behaviors accomplish? When Mrs. Smith becomes upset, how does Mary respond? Do her responses tend to make the situation better or worse? What are the top problems that need to be addressed for Mrs. Smith to be able to remain at home?

■ E: Enjoy the journey. Do Mrs. Smith and Mary have any shared values that have kept them together despite her disease? Can Mary articulate ways in which caring for her mom gives her life purpose or pleasure? Do the son-in-law and grandson help in Mrs. Smith's care, or are they resentful of the time and demands she places on them? As you come to know this family, what is it about them that you can appreciate?

In the next chapter, we see how the intake interview with Mrs. Smith and her daughter might evolve and how an A • B • C functional analysis can be developed to give you ideas for how to help this family. We also introduce a second case, that of Mrs. Flynn, to illustrate how the issues of obtaining consent and establishing rapport unfold in cases in which the care recipient is living alone and is referred without a proxy informant who can provide historical information.

4

DISCUSS CONCERNS RESPECTFULLY: ESTABLISHING CONSENT AND RAPPORT IN THE INITIAL INTERVIEW

Many prospective clients—individuals with dementia and their families alike—arrive at the initial appointment somewhat lost and apprehensive and without much of a preconceived notion as to what to expect. Regardless of when a diagnosis of dementia was made, how long family members have been caregivers, or how many services the family is already receiving, each time they meet with a new provider, families can have a sense of uncertainty about whether seeing you is necessary or whether it will be helpful to their current situation. The care recipients often arrive with fears about diminished functioning, compromised social status, loss of identity, and becoming a burden to others, as well as distrust regarding the role you will play in their future. Because of the prospective clients' uncertainty and apprehension concerning your potential services, the goal of the initial interview is to obtain informed consent and build rapport. When we tell our trainees to focus on making sure the clients will return for a second session, we are not joking. Generating hope and positive expectancies related to your services begins from the first time you meet.

ROME WASN'T BUILT IN A DAY

Clients come to our offices with a need to tell their story and with the expectation that we will help them figure out what to do next and as quickly as possible. This is understandable because getting a person with dementia to agree to a health care appointment can be challenging, and many people are struggling with transportation and financial pressures as well. However, quality dementia care cannot be rushed, and it is your task to balance your clients' desire to have their treatment expedited with the knowledge that all their problems do not need to be fixed immediately. If a diagnosis is recent and the care recipient is only mildly impaired, the development of long-term care plans and preventive strategies for the future requires careful deliberation and close knowledge of the care recipient's and the family's needs and wishes. Alternatively, by the time some families come to see you, conflict has escalated over the course of months and years; these caregivers may feel at the end of their rope and need you to help them take a deep breath and think through their future options clearly. Regardless of the level of urgency presented by the caregiver, we strongly advise you to take the intake session slowly. This first meeting will set the tone for what may be years or decades of follow-up consultations and care.

GETTING STARTED

For behavioral health care professionals, a typical initial session might take the following format: (a) welcome and session overview; (b) information gathering and building rapport; (c) informed consent process, including releases for the exchange of information with medical providers and dementia care agencies; (d) discussion of assessment and treatment options; and (e) homework and plans for the next session. In this chapter, we illustrate what these steps might look like, using the case of Mrs. Smith introduced in the Chapter 3, as well as a second case, that of Mrs. Flynn. Along the way, we highlight some additional clinical and logistic issues to consider, with a particular emphasis on demonstrating respect and acceptance of whatever the client and caregiver are each bringing to the session.

Welcome and Session Overview

The first few minutes with new clients are an opportunity for them to "size you up," to see whether you make them feel at ease and are someone whom they can trust with their concerns. This is particularly important for those with advancing dementia, who may rely more on nonverbal cues such as physical mannerisms, tone of voice, and affect rather than verbal content

TABLE 4.1
Sample Welcome or Session Overview

Health care professional	Comments
Hello, Mrs. Smith. Hello, Mary. Welcome. My name is Claudia. I am glad to greet you here at the Support Center. I know there's never enough time in a day, and travel is often cumbersome, so I'm happy you took the time to come and see us. Did you have any problems finding us? How was traffic? Did you use the highway, or did you come across town? Was parking easy?	• How you address your clients and ask them to address you can be important; first names are too informal for some older adults and surnames too formal for others. Invite them early on to express their preferences. • Inquiring about transportation concerns is one practical way to demonstrate your concern about the clients' needs. The caregiver's answers also provides insight into the level of difficulty he or she is experiencing providing routine instrumental care.
I would like to do several things today: I'd like to tell you a bit about me, so you can come to know me. At the same time, I'd also like to describe to you what I do here at the Support Center and what services we have to offer. Then I'd like to get to know a little about you. I'd like to talk to each of you separately about how you feel I can be most helpful to you. Then we'll all get back together and discuss where to go from here. After I have answered your questions, if you want to sign up for our services, you'll need to sign some documents similar to the ones you receive at a doctor's office. The paperwork will take a little time, and for that I apologize in advance. Does that sound okay to you? Do you have any questions about today?	• Depending on your business model or organizational system, families may have already completed much of the legal and financial and medical release paperwork before arriving in your office. If not, going over paperwork offers another opportunity to see how the client and caregiver work together and to get a sense of whether they are in agreement about the reasons for seeing you today.

as a basis for their interpersonal opinions. We feel strongly that it is best, whenever possible, to open the initial sessions with the caregiver and care recipient present together, as a way of communicating that both parties' perspectives and input are equally important. This also gives you an initial glimpse into the relationship between the caregiver and care recipient and their patterns of interaction. A sample opening session might look as is shown in Table 4.1.

Joint Versus Individual Sessions

As noted earlier, we usually prefer to meet with the caregiver and care recipient together at the first session. It is important, however, to also allow time to talk with each person separately. The initial session is an information and consent-gathering time. Unless the reason for the visit is extremely straightforward, it is not unusual for caregivers and care recipients to have widely differing opinions about what their problems are (or whether there are any problems at all). Consequently, it is both easier and more respectful to everyone concerned if you can talk briefly to each side in private. If there are multiple staff persons or trainees available, it may be possible to have different people meet separately with the caregiver and care recipient and then gather all parties together to confer before making treatment recommendations. Either way, we have found that the session goes most smoothly if you describe what you will be doing in your opening comments, so everyone knows what to expect.

It might seem that talking alone to a person with advanced dementia is a waste of precious clinical time, but in fact, that is not the case. It demonstrates to the care recipient that his or her opinion is important. It gives you a chance to conduct a brief cognitive screening to evaluate the severity of cognitive impairment. It allows you to assess for any mood or psychiatric symptoms and to observe whether they are the same or different from those reported by the caregiver or exhibited when the caregiver is in the room. In a relatively short period of time, you can build rapport with the care recipient and gain a wealth of behavioral observations that will help with your treatment recommendations. Similarly, the private interview with the caregiver allows him or her to elaborate on concerns he or she may have that cannot be freely discussed in the presence of the care recipient. It also gives you more uncensored access into the quality of the caregiving relationship. Is the caregiver dealing with additional extenuating circumstances that are adding to his or her burden? How is the caregiver's physical health and mood? Is he or she a good problem solver? Is there an outside support system? For some caregivers, this will be their first opportunity to "let it all out," and you will need to take care to not allow it to turn into an extended venting session that will keep the care recipient waiting and wondering what is being talked about.

Although in ideal situations, both caregiver and care recipient are able and willing to attend the intake appointment, in actual practice many caregivers attend the first appointment by themselves and do not schedule an intake for the care recipient. In other cases you, the provider, may prefer to meet only with the caregiver initially, on the basis of referral information you have been given. There are many reasons to see a caregiver alone. Some care recipients are so cognitively impaired and the referral question so specific to caregiving issues that only the caregiver needs to be seen. Some caregivers have had the experience that going to see health care professionals agitates the care recipient and creates conflict with the caregiver. Other caregivers do not know how to circumvent the care recipient's adamant refusal to leave the house or are embarrassed by their loved one's uncharacteristic behavior in public. Still others would like to treat behavioral health care sessions as their exclusive time away from the care recipient. It is important to inquire about these and other potential concerns in the initial intake session if the caregiver attends it alone. It is certainly possible to effectively treat caregivers without ever working with the care recipient. However, you should be aware that your assessment of the situation and what treatment options might be most helpful will remain limited by the caregiver's perspective, which in some cases can be quite narrow.

In the case of Mrs. Smith, the treating clinician originally planned to meet with Mary alone, given the apparently conflicted relationship between daughter and mother and Mrs. Smith's moderately severe cognitive impairment. The clinician was also concerned that because of Mrs. Smith's apparent fear of institutionalization and the fact that her dementia was advanced enough that she required 24-hr care, Mrs. Smith would not be able to participate in and consent to services. However, when we called to schedule an intake appointment, Mary said that she did not have access to respite and that she would need to bring Mrs. Smith to the appointment. Thus, the intake proceeded with both Mary and Mrs. Smith, who were privately interviewed in separate rooms after the initial greeting.

Information Gathering

Information gathering in dementia care has several stages. First of all, you need to give the clients an overview of some of the services you have to offer. They will have many specific questions, but your initial introduction can be simple, with as much inclusion of the care recipient as possible, such as in the following example:

> As you know, my name is Claudia. I work here at the Support Center. We provide services to persons who are older than 60 years of age and their families. Many of these clients have trouble with their memory. Whether they have trouble with their memory or not, we are interested in making sure that our clients have good relationships with friends and families. We are also interested in making sure that our clients have a generally good quality of life and are connected to community services. If you have concerns about your life, we could talk about them. For example, we can talk about how to get some help into the home, how to find a physician, what you can do about disagreements within your family, or what and how to plan for the future. However, we will not be able to do household chores for you or drive you. The center receives state and federal funding. This funding allows us to provide services, and nobody is turned away. [Turning first to the care recipient.] Which of our services might interest you?

The second stage of information gathering involves getting input from the caregiver and care recipient. This stage of information gathering takes several forms. First, you usually want the person with dementia to explain their situation and need for help, in their own words, as best they understand it. Even people with significant language impairments can be quite insightful and articulate about their difficulties when given an unpressured opportunity to express themselves. Second, information gathering involves talking with proxy informants: the primary caregiver, as well as any other family, friends, or health care professionals who may have information and insight that is pertinent to your evaluation and care for the client. Last, we gather considerable information from persons with dementia simply by observing their interactions with us and with other people. Interviewing cognitively impaired persons requires a delicate balance between knowing when it is time to "get the facts" and when it is time to step back and focus on redirecting the client into some form of meaningful engagement just for its own sake. This balancing act shifts over time as dementia progresses, with more of an emphasis on the fact gathering and dialogue in early stages of disease and a greater reliance on proxies and interpersonal engagement later on. In our practice, we frequently see clients who are diagnosed with early onset Alzheimer's initially in their 50s and continue to be followed for many years. In other cases, adult children may first begin seeing you with concerns about one parent, then continue over the years under your care as the other parent also starts to need help. The establishment of a solid and trusting working relationship early on—through discussions of the diagnosis, concerns, and individual needs for assistance—makes it possible for us to conduct assessments and provide services later on, when the person might be more suspicious of health care providers. In general, taking the time to come to know your clients, their values, and their preferences will help you weigh and explore treatment options later. It will enable you to become an effective advocate and a voice for your clients as decline progresses.

Building Rapport

Whether clients decide that they will be part of this collaborative relationship depends in large part on your rapport-building skills, including the nonverbal impression you make at this first session. As you are reading this book, take a minute and check in with yourself: How are you sitting? Are your legs crossed and tense, or are you relaxed? Is your back straight, or are you slouching? Is your brow furrowed as you are reading? Are the corners of your mouth turned down or relaxed in a neutral position or a half smile? Is there tension in your shoulders? Are you pulling them up? What might an outside observer surmise about you? As we pointed out earlier, individuals with dementia who are losing their spoken language ability often attend to your facial expression, voice properties, and physical demeanor to compensate for their losses. We tell both our trainees and caregivers to assume care recipients can read their subtle shifts in emotions like an open book, even though they might have lost the ability to make sense of, appropriately address, or cope with a particular emotion. Consequently, basic good clinical interviewing skills are of exaggerated importance when you work with cognitively impaired clients. Try to achieve a warm style and appear relaxed, confident, and empathic. Do not allow the caregiver and the care recipient (or multiple caregivers in the intake session) to complain about or argue with each other, lest the individual with dementia come to associate your office with conflict. Slow down. Be respectful and courteous.

Practicing POLITE Communication

In her previous guide for families, McCurry (2006) used the acronym POLITE to describe effective communication with individuals with moderate to severe dementia. This acronym, elaborated in Exhibit 4.1, is also useful for health care providers.

We should make one final note about rapport building. In addition to being aware of your own nonverbal communication, it is equally important to attend to nonverbal cues from your cognitively impaired clients. For those who are having increasing difficulty with verbal self-expression, physical gestures, body agitation, facial grimaces or smiles, and vocal volume become important tools for letting other people know how they are feeling. Dr. Steve Albert at University of Pittsburgh has said that one of the last functions a person with advanced dementia loses is the ability to know whether something is pleasing or not (Albert et al. 1996).[1] In this respect, persons with dementia are genuine; in the words of the famous pop song, "What you see is what you get." This lack of guile and spontaneous expression of inner experience, particularly in more advanced stages of the disease, led one caregiver to tell us, "It is like being able to look into my wife's very soul." The alert health care professional will take advantage of this to gather invaluable information about how what he or she is saying and doing is being received by the client and also about the client's preferences, which will be important if you are going to provide effective treatment. Table 4.2 shows how the information-gathering and rapport-building process went with Mrs. Smith and Mary at their intake visit and how this might lead to a tentative treatment plan.

---

[1]For persons interested in Dr. Albert's approach to using observable behaviors such as facial and body expressions to assess quality of life in persons unable to articulate their inner experiences, see Albert et al. (1996). All studies on conditioning without awareness (i.e., overt versus covert or explicit versus implicit knowing), including those cited earlier, rely on the ability of events to affect behavior even when a person is not able to describe or verbally respond to them anymore.

EXHIBIT 4.1
POLITE Communication

Patience	Assume that individuals with dementia, like everyone else, appreciate conversations. Slow down your pace to meet the abilities of the person with dementia. If necessary, use shorter sentences. Many providers fall into a question–answer trap; instead, ask open-ended questions and wait for answers. Although individuals with dementia might not remember the content of the conversation, they will remember its style; you cannot build rapport through what the other person perceives to be interrogation. If the person with dementia is unable to answer an open-ended question, introduce choices.
Organization	Not knowing "what is next" is a constant and gnawing concern for individuals with dementia. Make reminder calls to clients, if appropriate. Include a prompt to make sure that the care recipient has access to his or her usual prosthetic devices (e.g., eye glasses, hearing aids, dentures) during the appointment. Schedule appointments so as to avoid prolonged waiting periods because these can increase client apprehension and agitation. Provide distractions in the waiting room and an easily accessible and findable restroom.
Laughter	Engage in self-disclosure through story-telling to give clients a "feel" for you. Smile frequently, and laugh with the person with dementia to put him or her at ease. If language skills are compromised, then you will set the mood, and the person with dementia usually matches it. People with severe dementia will appreciate an opportunity to engage in smiling, laughing, and simple conversation with you.
Individualization	No two individuals (with or without dementia) are alike. Beware of ageist or disability-related terminology such as "the elderly" or "the demented"; take time to know the person, his or her history, dreams, and fears. Individualize your services and be creative: What might be a good solution for one person with dementia may be a bad fit for another. When a person reports upset, anger, and so forth, do not be dismissive. For example, if a person reports that her family will abandon her in a nursing home, do not answer, "Of course not. You shouldn't feel this way after all your family has done." Rather say, "It sounds like you are really worried about this." Then distract or address the concerns, depending on a person's level of cognitive impairment.
Tone of voice	Cultivate a style that communicates respect and warmth. Avoid language or intonations that might be construed as patronizing or parental. Notice if you speak louder than necessary when the client is slow to respond. Refrain from lecturing; even if you "know best" what a client needs, keep it to yourself, at least for the moment. Find out what the client has tried in the past and what he finds feasible and workable. Together, explore multiple courses of action and then collaborate with the client to weigh options. Offer praise when it is sincere. Ask yourself: Would I want to be talked to this way?
Eye contact	Even if you know that the person with dementia does not understand the specific content of conversation, continue frequent eye contact and include him or her in the conversation with direct smiles and nods. If a person has a hearing impairment, establish eye contact while addressing the person to be sure of her attention. Sit at the same level as the client rather than talking down to him or her.

Note. Clinicians new to work with cognitively impaired individuals sometimes find themselves at a loss for how to elicit information about clients' personal preferences and values. In such cases, the Quality of Life-Alzheimer's Disease (Logsdon, Gibbons, McCurry, & Teri, 1999) can be a useful tool for structuring the first interview. When administered to the caregiver as well as the care recipient, the clinician can also gather useful information regarding differences in how the two parties view their situation, which may influence treatment planning. Adapted from *When a Family Member Has Dementia: Steps to Becoming a Resilient Caregiver,* by S. M. McCurry, 2006. Copyright 2006 by Praeger Publishers. Reproduced with permission of ABC-CLIO, LLC.

TABLE 4.2
Mrs. Smith's Information Gathering Process

Clinician observations	Comments
When Mrs. Smith and Mary arrived at the clinic, Mary seemed upset. Her face was reddened, her lips pressed together, and the corners of her mouth turned down. Mrs. Smith, who was nicely dressed, was quietly trailing behind. She did not seem to have trouble ambulating. Mother and daughter did not talk to each other while waiting. After the initial welcome, Mrs. Smith willingly accompanied a staff member into a second treatment room.	• On entering the clinic, Mrs. Smith was calm. She offered no resistance to following a staff person to a separate room. This suggests that there may be other situational activators for the angry and agitated behaviors described in Mrs. Smith's referral notes.
Mary told her therapist that before the appointment, Mrs. Smith had announced: "I'm not going with her. I'm not going to be part of this thing . . . this hostile takeover." Mary became Mrs. Smith's guardian almost 2 years ago, after Mrs. Smith had refused to stop driving. Mary has been overseeing Mrs. Smith's medical, legal, financial, and personal care needs since that time. She brought a copy of the order for guardianship with her. Mary said that Mrs. Smith had been physically abused as a child and had subsequently been abusive to Mary as a child. It quickly became evident that Mary tended to attribute her mother's difficult behaviors to "intention" and "part of her personality" rather than to her profound cognitive deficits.	• Mary is clearly distressed and emotionally distant from her mom. The history she provided suggests that relationship problems between them are long-standing. • Despite their differences, Mary has assumed responsibility for her mother's care for almost 2 years, indicating a real commitment to helping Mrs. Smith. • Mary needs some basic dementia education, including communication training because she relies heavily on reasoning and verbal persuasion to influence Mrs. Smith. We should follow up on whether marital or family counseling is indicated given the shared living arrangement. Additional community resource referral needs should also be examined.
Meanwhile, in the separate room, Mrs. Smith was initially fearful and repeatedly expressed concern that plans were being made to institutionalize her or take away her legal rights. However, as she talked with the psychologist and student trainee, she became pleasant and described herself as a person who "stands up for others," including animals. She was delighted to meet a resident therapy dog ("Spot") who would be able to be with her in any future visits to the clinic. Despite obvious memory and word-finding difficulties, Mrs. Smith smiled frequently, had a sense of humor, conversed readily, and offered the student her own chair to sit in.	• Mrs. Smith is pleasant and cooperative as long as she is approached in a respectful and dignified way. • She particularly dislikes being told what to do (without offering her a choice or asking permission) and being "babied" (providing assistance with self-care). She reacts strongly to nonverbal facial cues (positive or negative). • Mrs. Smith's history of abuse, involuntary hospitalizations, and multiple changes in living situation may contribute to her suspiciousness and distrust. When she feels safe, she exhibits considerable intact social skills.

DISCUSS CONCERNS RESPECTFULLY   59

TABLE 4.3
Overview of Steps in the A • B • Cs for Mrs. Smith

Activators	Mrs. Smith's behaviors	Consequences
Mary asking Mrs. Smith to take her medications Mary talking about her mom to other people in the room Mary telling Mrs. Smith what clothes to wear People physically trying to control Mrs. Smith's actions Mary providing personal care Mary looking angry or upset	Refusing to accept help with personal care Unsafe self-directed behaviors (driving, cooking) Verbal (accusing) and physical (hitting, shoving, scratching, pushing) behavior Wandering	Mary tries to reason with her mother and to convince her to stop acting this way. Mary exhibits angry and frustrated tone of voice, body language, and facial expression. Mary labels her mother's actions as "aggressive."
Broader psychosocial context: Family moving in with Mrs. Smith following discharge from residential care and multiple psychiatric hospitalizations History of Mrs. Smith being both abusive and helpful to Mary at different times in the past Mrs. Smith's vision (cataracts) Good relationships between Mrs. Smith and professional caregivers	*Gather a behavioral history:* Gradual worsening in behavior over time Abrupt changes with major losses (e.g., taking car away) and moves (hospitalizations, moving in with daughter)	*Pleasant events for Mrs. Smith:* Choice, animals, chocolate, TV, friendly conversations, having a nice appearance, being talked to respectfully

Conducting a Functional Analysis

Following the intake interviews with Mrs. Smith and Mary, you now have sufficient information to start the process of conducting a functional analysis of Mrs. Smith's case. Table 4.3 shows some of the activators and consequences that were discovered during their first visit. As you look at these, you might consider how they could lead to recommendations for interventions with Mrs. Smith and her daughter. What other information would you like to know?

Prior to the first appointment, the clinician had intended to meet only with Mary because she had legal guardianship and the clinician was con-

cerned that Mrs. Smith would be unable to give her consent for, or participate in, treatment at the clinic. After talking with Mrs. Smith privately, however, it became clear that she would also assent to periodic visits to the clinic
so long as she perceived that she was being treated with respect, was given
limited and safe access to choices, and did not have her deficits pointed out
to her. She was cooperative with requests for help (e.g., "Can you help me
take your blood pressure?") and easily distracted by the presence of an animal.
All future visits were scheduled to be conducted with Mrs. Smith and Mary
seen separately. Mrs. Smith was invited to "help out" the more physically disabled participants at the senior adult day program and she integrated well into
the group. Mary was coached in a variety of dementia communication and
behavior management skills through a combination of six individual and
caregiver group sessions. She was also provided with information about alternative community services and residential care options that might be utilized
as Mrs. Smith's condition continued to progress.

Obtaining Informed Consent

Although Mrs. Smith did assent to the treatment her guardian daughter was seeking, things are not always so easy. It is not rare for family members to want desperately to get a parent or spouse evaluated and treated for
possible dementia and for that parent or spouse to adamantly refuse. We
sometimes forget that older adults, including those with dementia, have as
much right to make decisions frowned on by other people as do their (often
younger) caregivers. In recent years, there has been a great deal of discussion
about the ethics of treating cognitively impaired individuals (Karlawish,
2008; Kim et al., 2009) and the implications for clinical practice with these
clients. How does dementia affect the ability of clients to judge whether or
not they need help? How can we both protect clients' rights to make their
own decisions but also protect them from the adverse effects of bad decisions
they might make because they cannot think through the consequences of
their actions? Last, how can we be certain that those who do agree to treatment in our office do so with real understanding of what they are agreeing to?

Informed consent to accept or refuse services is based on the capacity to
make a voluntary choice and presupposes the integration of sufficient information to choose in an informed manner. As defined by Grisso and Appelbaum
(1998), *informed consent* means that care recipients have: (a) the ability to
express a choice; (b) the ability to understand information relevant to treatment decision making; (c) the ability to appreciate the significance of that
information for one's own situation, especially concerning one's illness and the
probable consequences of one's treatment options; and (d) the ability to reason with relevant information so as to engage in a logical process of weighing

treatment options.[2] Neither a dementia diagnosis nor standardized test scores—especially if they are in the mildly to moderately impaired range—indicate whether a person is able to voluntarily and fully consent to your services. In most cases, a formal judicial evaluation of global competency will not have been conducted, so you will have to carefully assess individuals' understanding of the current situation to determine whether they are capable of choosing or declining your services in an informed and voluntary manner.

Probes to Ascertain Understanding

One of the first steps in evaluating a care recipient's capacity to consent to treatment is to talk with the caregiver. The caregiver will often know whether the care recipient is able to answer in a content-appropriate fashion and has the decisional capacity to sign up for services. If a person has already been given a diagnosis of dementia, a durable health care power of attorney may have been executed. Each state has laws pertaining to when previously designated attorneys-in-fact are able to stand in as proxy decision makers and the extent and the limits of durable health care powers of attorney. Familiarize yourself with the statutes of your state. When informed consent is given by proxy, the person with dementia might still be able to assent to services, give permission for assessment, and indicate whether he or she would like to return for a second appointment with you.

In other cases, a person's cognitive symptoms may be quite mild and the caregiver may not know whether the care recipient has dementia or not. Many individuals with even moderate cognitive impairment retain excellent social skills and are able to read social cues. They might be able to nod agreement or shake their head in disapproval at the appropriate time; they might be able to carry on small talk, give advice in the form of adages, and generally compensate for declining problem-solving ability with social graces. In this situation, you need to gently probe whether the care recipient is able to produce some of the information you provided in a short, precursory statement. If a care recipient is, after your introduction, able to specify that you work with older adults, work on improving relationships, and are associated with the university, there is a good chance that he will be able to participate in informed consent. If he is willing to consent to treatment, you should invite the client to also sign standard releases for the exchange of information between you and other providers (e.g., primary care physician, neurologist, psychiatrist) who are involved in other aspects of the client's care.

---

[2]For further guidance on assessing capacity and informed consent, see http://www.apa.org/pi/aging/programs/assessment/capacity-psychologist-handbook.pdf.

When Help Is Needed but Not Wanted

It is much easier to ascertain on the basis of a clinical interview whether a person is able to give consent than it is to figure out whether an unwillingness to consent is done with full understanding and whether action needs to be taken against a person's stated wishes. Many caregivers are unclear about the etiology of the symptoms they are observing. Is Mom acting this way because she is still grieving over Dad's death? Grandpa has always been stubborn and has always had a temper; is he just getting more cantankerous with age? For persons who are living independently and resisting medical evaluation or care, the law tends to favor protecting the autonomy of the individual unless there is a demonstrable danger to self or others. If the person is in real danger and has not formally named an attorney-in-fact, then the initiation of a financial conservator or guardianship procedure may become necessary. This is not a swift or a simple process, and you will be of great help to your clients if you have a referral sheet with a list of respected elder law attorneys nearby. Note that guardianship or conservatorship also may be needed instead of an attorney-in-fact when the care recipient is prone toward uncharacteristic decisions that potentially put him or her in harm's way, such as impulsively getting on a Greyhound bus and taking a cross-country trip, without goals, detailed plans, a change of clothes, or money. Once guardianship proceedings begin, the care recipient will not be able to receive services until his or her legal consent status has been formalized within the judicial system.

The most difficult cases can be those referrals that come to you from outside sources rather than from family caregivers. One of us (Claudia) receives many referrals from Elder Protective Services in her clinical practice (sometimes up to 40% of her case load). In some situations, it is the caregivers who are referred because they are suspected of neglect, exploitation, or abuse of the care recipient. Although most health care services are confidential and protected by federal privacy law (i.e., the Health Insurance Portability and Accountability Act), as mandated reporters you also need to make sure that these referred caregiver clients, in addition to being informed about the terms of your services, have a full understanding of the conditions under which you will be required to break confidentiality. In other situations, the outside referral is for potentially vulnerable older adults, particularly those who are living alone, who come to the attention of an astute neighbor or business/community representative who notices the older adult is having trouble. Consider the following case of Mrs. Flynn.

CASE 2. MRS. FLYNN: HELPING INDIVIDUALS WHO LIVE ALONE

Mrs. Flynn is a 90-year-old woman who lives alone with her cockatiel, Smokey, in her two-story home. She does not have any children or living relatives. Recently, workers from the electricity company made a call to Mrs. Flynn to shut off the electricity after she had failed to pay her bills for 6 months. When the workers knocked on the door, Mrs. Flynn readily invited them into her home. Mrs. Flynn's appearance was unremarkable: She was well groomed and dressed. She wore hearing aids in both of her ears. Her home was clean and tidy and so was the birdcage. Smokey had fresh food and water. Mrs. Flynn seemed unaware that her bills had not been paid. The workers noticed that she did not know what month or year it was and that she failed to understand that her behavior had led to their presence. Mrs. Flynn repeatedly directed the workers to her collection of figurines on the shelves, pointed out how often they had to be dusted, and said she could manage them well on her own. Whenever the workers reintroduced the issue of unpaid bills and the company's request to shut off her electricity, Mrs. Flynn reverted to talking about the effort involved in keeping up her figurine collection. One of the workers asked to make a call from Mrs. Flynn's phone and noticed that the phone line was dead. Mrs. Flynn said that she had had trouble with her phone for a while. The workers postponed shutting off the electricity and reported their observations to the local Elder Protective Services unit. After conducting an initial assessment during which immediate danger to self was ruled out and payment of outstanding bills through a financial assistance program was arranged, Elder Protective Services referred the case to you. Mrs. Flynn consented to attend an appointment with you.

As with the case of Mrs. Smith, we can use the DANCE principles and principles of functional analysis to begin to conceptualize the case. Think about other questions you would have in mind prior to meeting with Mrs. Flynn for the first time.

- D: Discuss concerns respectfully. Mrs. Flynn is still living independently. Although she is having difficulty paying her bills, in other areas (i.e., her personal appearance, upkeep of the home and bird cage) she seems to be functioning well. Does Mrs. Flynn understand the reason for her referral to you? Does she perceive that she has any need for assistance? Do you think she is capable of giving informed consent for evaluation and treatment? Does she have a designated power of attorney? If not, should a public guardian appointed?
- A: Ameliorate excess disability. When was the last time Mrs. Flynn had a thorough medical examination? Does she have any known comorbidities that place her at risk of cognitive decline? What medications does she take, and has she been taking them properly? Can we determine whether Mrs. Flynn's decline has been sudden or gradual?
- N: Nurture the dyad. What aspects of her current lifestyle are important to Mrs. Flynn? How long has she been living alone?

TABLE 4.4
Overview of Steps in the A • B • Cs for Mrs. Flynn

Activators	Behaviors	Consequences
Living alone without assistance or family supervision	Disoriented to date	Phone line was disconnected; power about to be turned off.
Unknown medical, behavioral, psychosocial history at this time	Paying her bills late	Workers unsuccessfully tried to talk to her about the unpaid bills.
	Inviting strangers into her home	
	Answering utility workers' questions about her home service inappropriately	
	Repeated conversation about context-inappropriate topics	Electrical company contacted Elder Protective Services (EPS).
Broader psychosocial context: Referral from EPS sets stage for initiation of proceedings for public guardianship, if needed.	*Gather a behavioral history:* Unknown.	*Pleasant events for Mrs. Flynn:* Smokey, the cockatiel; attending to her figurines

Does she have any family, neighbors, or friends who could provide additional background information and assist in overseeing her independent living? Is she happy with her current living arrangement? Would she enjoy living in a smaller home or around other people?

- C: Create contextual solutions. It is currently unknown whether Mrs. Flynn is experiencing any changes in her mood or behavior other than those related to memory, orientation, and comprehension of complex information leading to her failure to stay current with household bills (see Table 4.4). What other instrumental activities of daily living might also be suffering in Mrs. Flynn's life and need investigation? How can you gather this information in the absence of a reliable proxy informant?
- E: Enjoy the journey. Other than her pet cockatiel, what does Mrs. Flynn have in her daily life that brings her satisfaction and pleasure? Does she have other health care providers whom she trusts and feels close to? How can you build on her cognitive and social strengths to assist her long-term planning?

In the next chapter, readers see how to begin the assessment and treatment process with vulnerable older adults like Mrs. Flynn who are living alone and experiencing cognitive decline. We also introduce a third case, that of Mrs. Puttani, to illustrate how the issues of sensory loss and medical morbidity can impact quality of life for severely cognitively impaired residents living in skilled nursing care facilities.

5

AMELIORATE EXCESS DISABILITY: TREATING SENSORY LOSS AND COMORBIDITIES

In the previous chapters, we described how to use the DANCE principles and functional analysis to generate hypotheses about the psychosocial factors contributing to changes in your clients' mood and behavior. In Mrs. Smith's case, we saw that her agitation increased when she was treated disrespectfully or "bossed around" by caregivers who were trying to offer much-needed assistance with personal care. With Mrs. Flynn, living alone placed her at risk of personal harm and exploitation because she could no longer remember to pay her bills or to be cautious about opening her door to strangers. In this chapter, we review some of the common physical factors that are often part of clients' psychosocial context and that can worsen cognitive impairment and exacerbate mood and behavioral changes in persons with dementia.

EXCESS DISABILITY IN DEMENTIA

Think about the last time you had a "bad day," perhaps because of a gnawing headache or lack of sleep the night before. Even though you were not feeling "up to par," chances are that you functioned just fine and any ill effects on your interactions with other people were subtle and barely noticeable.

However, what would happen if in addition to your headache, you had a secondary sinus infection or a bad back sprain? Would you not be more likely to be distracted or irritable or prone to make mistakes on the job? This is what we mean when we talk about excess disability: The person with dementia is doing worse than predicted by the dementing disease alone because something else is going on. The list of things that might go wrong is long. It spans from unmanaged chronic illnesses that the client may have lived with for years, to uncorrected sensory loss, to acute anxiety and depression. Regardless of the particular concurrent problem, it will add additional burden to a person who is already struggling with cognitive impairment.

A colleague, Dr. Linda Teri, has compared the treatment of excess disability in dementia to a man on crutches who is trying to walk dragging a heavy ball and chain that is tied to one leg (Reifler, Larson, & Teri, 1987). We may not be able to solve the problem that originally made the man need crutches, but if we can remove the ball and chain he is going to move around a lot more easily. We may not be able to cure dementia, but if we can treat our clients' additional concurrent, or comorbid problems, they will be able to function better, regardless of their stage of disease. Sometimes, challenging dementia-related behaviors "miraculously" disappear when pain and discomfort are effectively treated. In fact, rather than being a true problem, seemingly difficult behaviors can actually serve to draw needed attention to the care recipient, alerting caregivers to serious, even life-threatening, conditions such as a urinary tract or a prostate infection, chronic pain, constipation, pneumonia, or cancer. Because of the important and sometimes dramatic effects of correcting excess disability, this chapter is dedicated to ruling it out. This is where a big chunk of your contextual detective work comes into play.

WHY IS IT DETECTIVE WORK?

Many clients with dementia are unable to tell you or their caregivers when something is physically or emotionally wrong with them. This is surprising to many of our trainees. Shouldn't the care recipient be able to tell you that he or she has a pain in his or her chest? Shouldn't even someone with memory problems know how he or she feels right now?

Although it seems plausible that a person should find it easier to express what is going on inside of him than to talk about external events, this is not always the case. Linguists have pointed out that for all humans, subtle emotions and inner experiences are better communicated through nonverbal cues than by spoken language (Pinker & Bloom, 1990). Indeed, teaching children to describe even not-so-subtle internal events, such as headaches or tummy aches, is a prolonged and complicated process during which parents rely on observable collaterals to figure out what is going on. Is the child pale? Does she hold her forehead? Did he eat less for breakfast and seem subdued? As typically developing children get older, we expect them to be able to tell us what is wrong without parental prompting, based on their internal stimulation alone. Over time, we tend to forget that describing physiological and psychological internal states is a verbal skill that took us years to learn.

It is important to remember in your work with individuals with dementia that their ability to express internal states or emotions can be fragile and fickle. Some persons who are capable of enjoying small talk or reminiscences are completely unable to tell you when something feels uncomfortable. Some people need additional prompts to be able to describe what is going on inside, whether it is nausea, a migraine headache, heartburn, dizziness, or fear. Verbal aphasia may cause them to recognize the correct condition if it is named, but they may be unable to describe it on their own. Visual cues such as pointing to the head or stomach and grimacing may be more evocative than verbal queries. We do not mean to imply that individuals with dementia become childlike or lose their personal histories and preferences. Instead, we think of self-reporting as another complex chain of steps—such as taking a shower or setting a pendulum clock—that has broken down or become unreliable. Like other overlearned activities of daily living affected by dementia, self-report is a skill that we all take for granted but that can be lost. For this reason, health professionals need to be especially alert and always on the lookout for nonverbal cues, including unusual or disruptive behaviors that say what words cannot.

RULING OUT EXCESS DISABILITY STEP-BY-STEP

Our clinical practice has confirmed Dr. Hussian's (1981) rule of thumb: If a behavioral or affective problem has emerged abruptly and is severe enough to be brought to your attention, it probably is not a direct result of the dementing disorder. Whenever a person presents with affective or behavioral problems and a notable decline in cognitive functioning, an evaluation for possible comorbid conditions should always be conducted. The following step-by-step considerations follow recommendations by the American Academy of Neurology, Ethics, and Humanities Subcommittee (1996) for evaluating common causes of excess disability in dementia.

1. Ruling Out Decrements in Typical Physical Functioning

A variety of changes in physical status can influence the mood and behavior of older adults, particularly those with cognitive impairment. Many of these status changes are so commonplace they are easy to overlook, but the consequences of doing so can be serious or even life threatening.

Nutrition

What do your clients eat? This is an important question because many people with dementia lose interest in food. Potential changes in olfactory, gustatory, visual, tactile, and auditory functioning may result in food not smelling, tasting, looking, feeling, or sounding as appetizing or stimulating as it once did. This can lead to multiple downstream health consequences. For example, a medical referral for Mrs. Flynn revealed that she had a vitamin B_{12} deficiency that could have contributed to her cognitive impairment. She did not recall when she had last eaten. Although her housekeeping seemed immaculate, an inspection of her refrigerator revealed many expired and spoilt food items, putting Mrs. Flynn at risk of food-borne illnesses.

However, when food aroma, taste, texture, appearance, and social cues associated with eating are enhanced, people may rediscover their appetites. Although undernutrition and unintentional weight loss are well-known concerns for older people living in long-term care (Salva et al., 2009), our experience has been that many people with dementia rally, gain weight, and become physically stronger after moving into a more social setting. Individuals who enjoy the communal aspects of meals and appreciate being offered a range of food choices could especially benefit from the dining routines provided by many residential care facilities.

Hydration

Are your clients drinking enough water? Like malnutrition, dehydration is a major risk factor for increased confusion. Because of the changes in sensory functioning described earlier as well as age-related changes in water regulation, many people with dementia are particular about fluids. For example, Mrs. Smith's daughter Mary reported that her mother never answered yes when offered fluids. However, if Mary put a glass of water into her mother's hand, she would drink it. Because a lack of perceived thirst is typical, many people benefit from measured, bottled fluids, with the task to empty the bottle by a certain time. The amount of fluids to ingest depends on the physician's recommendations and environmental circumstances. For example, in Claudia's practice in Nevada, preventing dehydration is a top priority. In high temperatures, even normal walking can lead to water depletion at rates of about 1.5 liters per hour, and at altitudes over 6,000 ft people exhale and perspire twice as much moisture as at sea level. Nevada's high desert thus puts care recipients at risk of dehydration. Because many care recipients outright refuse liquids, problem solving is part of the daily routine. Offering liquids in different forms can increase consumption; some individuals will only accept and enjoy iced water or lemon water, whereas others refuse categorically to drink water presented in any form. In the latter case, you can prompt caregivers to collaborate with physicians and establish a list of alternative fluids, such as finely ground ice chips, carbonated water, decaffeinated coffee and teas, or nonfat milk.

Sleep

What is your client's sleep schedule? Does she have a daily routine with consistent bed and rising times? Is he spending long periods of time during the day napping or being physically inactive? Chronic sleep deprivation undermines caregiver and care recipient physiological and psychological well-being, decreases stress tolerance and immune function, contributes to premature care recipient institutionalization, and is associated with increased mortality risk. The neuronal changes found in Alzheimer's disease and other dementias disrupt 24-hr circadian temperature, hormonal, and rest–activity patterns, making it increasingly difficult for family caregivers to hold care recipients to routines that are most conducive to nighttime sleep. Many common age-related health conditions, including primary sleep disorders (e.g., sleep apnea), cardiac and lung disease, arthritis pain, prostate disease, and medications used to treat them can further affect sleep quality and routines. The A • B • Cs are useful for identifying medical, environmental, and behavioral activators for nighttime awakenings in persons with dementia (for more about this, see Chapter 7). There is also growing evidence that nonpharmacological strategies known to improve the sleep of adults without dementia diagnoses, such as reducing time in bed, increasing light exposure and exercise or social activation, can improve sleep in cognitively impaired individuals as well.[1]

An alternative treatment approach is to accept the consequences of a deteriorating circadian system and allow persons with dementia to set their

---

[1]A growing literature exists on the biology underlying irregular sleep–wake rhythms in cognitively impaired older adults and on nonpharmacological interventions that can improve sleep in both institutional and community-based settings. The latter are significant because sleep problems are highly prevalent in persons with dementia (Vitiello & Borson, 2001), and to date, there are no clinical trials demonstrating the safety and efficacy of any sedating medications to treat them. Individuals interested in learning more about the neurophysiology of sleep in dementia might refer to Harper et al. (2005); Hatfield, Herbert, van Someren, Hodges, and Hastings (2004); or Lee, Friedland, Whitehouse, and Woo (2004). For information on nonpharmacological treatments pertinent to older adults with dementia, see reviews by Bloom et al. (2009); Cole and Richards (2006); Martin and Ancoli-Israel (2008); McCurry, Reynolds, Ancoli-Israel, Teri, and Vitiello (2000); Sack et al. (2007), or Terman (2007).

On a related note, caregiver sleep is also an issue for many dyads and can exist independent of sleep disturbances in the care recipient. Although some of the risk factors and treatment options overlap with those for cognitively impaired individuals, sleep disturbances in caregivers deserve their own careful contextual assessment and problem solving to address effectively (McCurry, Gibbons, Logsdon, Vitiello, & Teri, 2009; McCurry, Logsdon, Teri, & Vitiello, 2007).

own sleep–wake schedules. This will generally not work for individuals who are still living in the community with family caregivers who can become exhausted caring for someone who sleeps all day and is up all night. However, some long-term care facilities are designed to accommodate residents who have day–night reversals in sleep–wake patterns or who need to sleep in multiple small bouts throughout a 24-hr period. Recently, outpatient adult day programs that are open only at night for those persons with intractable nocturnal sleep problems are becoming available, with reported good success (Buckley & Estrin, 2009).

Bowel and Urinary Functioning

Although its discussion may be embarrassing for individuals with dementia and their families, one cannot underestimate the effects of optimized bowel and urinary functioning on quality of life. Constipation or impaction as well as urinary retention may result in discomfort that rises to the level of excruciating pain. A person with dementia who experiences such a noxious event may seem delirious and engage in highly unusual behaviors (e.g., striking others, losing verbal coherence, moving furniture out of his room). Urinary retention can also lead to chronic urinary tract infections and, subsequently, kidney damage. Monitoring regular bowel movements and urination is thus important.

Fecal and urinary incontinence are also social stressors. Frequently, family relationships deteriorate when a spouse or adult child begins to provide continence care, from wiping after bowel movements to changing adult briefs. Most cultures teach people to be mortified to share with others these most private and taboo experiences, so not surprisingly, continence care is often the functional activator of care recipient self-protective behaviors such as hitting and pushing away. Once incontinence sets in, many families do not consult medical specialists because laypeople tend to believe that dementia and incontinence go hand-in-hand. Contrary to this common belief, however, there is no one-to-one correlation of dementia with incontinence; incontinence happens for a range of reasons and takes many different forms. Sometimes incontinence is reversible, even when a dementia diagnosis is present. Consequently, a medical incontinence assessment is necessary.

In advancing dementia, many people still detect the urge to urinate or defecate but cannot follow through on the next step: finding a toilet or, even if it is found, properly sitting down on it or standing close enough to urinate into it. Combined with an inability to describe one's internal experiences, a person may be in "sensation limbo." He or she may feel the strong urge to do "something," without being able to take any goal-directed or purposeful action and without being able to express any urgent need. Restlessness is but one of the consequences; behavior interpreted as "aggressive," such as pushing residents out of the way; exposing one's genitals; or entering other residents' rooms and relieving oneself there may also result. Toileting schedules, arranged in collaboration with the treating physician, are an excellent preventive tool for such understandable restlessness and confused, albeit desperate, action. Taking the person to the bathroom at predetermined intervals (usually every 3 or 4 hr) can spare the care recipient and his or her caregiver much aggravation.

Another common problem is the disposing of adult continence care items. We have pointed to the highly embarrassing nature of incontinence and the preserved sensitivity to social cues in dementia. Even when a person is fully incontinent of bladder, he or she may still use the restroom once in a while. Thus, it is not uncommon that individuals with urinary incontinence will remove their adult briefs while using the restroom and then not be able to determine what to do next. Used continence care items show up in cutlery drawers, under beds, in closets, up shirtsleeves, and in pockets and handbags and fish tanks. Although these disposal methods are often viewed as deliberately provocative by caregivers and staff, they are simply evidence of a client's preserved social patterns of behavior (appropriate embarrassment and not wanting to be scolded), combined with confusion and inability to ask for the disposal bin. Here again, a regular toileting schedule may eradicate the problem. In addition, we recommend that staff or family members always welcome the presentation of used continence care materials, rather than questioning the care recipient's decision to take them off.

Baseline Activity Level

How physically active are you in your life at present? Do you exercise? How much of the day do you spend on your feet? Regardless of whether your clients are octogenarians or belong to the baby boomer generation, many of them have extensive and sometimes intensive histories of physical activity. Among our clients were enthusiastic golfers who walked the golf course daily for 2 decades, marathon runners whose last finished race was but 5 years in the past, and soccer players trained to effortlessly endure 90 min of running, dribbling, kicking, and jumping. Some behaviors that are labeled "restlessness" or "wandering" simply reflect a shift from a lifetime of high activity to low. Lack of physical exercise and boredom may also lead to excessive daytime sleeping with resulting nighttime wakefulness. Knowledge of your client's baseline activity level is helpful in arranging long-term care plans that anticipate his or her need to be physically active and thereby prevent motoric restlessness or its escalation into agitation.

Case Example of Decrements in Typical Physical Functioning: Mrs. Smith

In the referral information and intake visit described earlier for our first case, Mrs. Smith, we learned that resistance to being told what to do, particularly with regard to personal care, was a common activator to many of

TABLE 5.1
More Refined A • B • Cs for Mrs. Smith

Activators	Mrs. Smith's behaviors	Consequences
Mary providing personal care, as follows: • Mary prompting Mrs. Smith to wear her "diapers" • Mary telling Mrs. Smith she needed to check her diaper • Mary pulling Mrs. Smith's pants down to check for wetness • Mary commenting on "smelling poo"	Hitting, shoving, scratching, pushing	Immediate consequences: • Mary tries to reason with her mother and to convince her to stop acting this way. • Mary exhibits angry or frustrated tone of voice, body language, and facial expression. • Mary ceases her efforts to provide continence care to her mom. Long-term consequences: • Mary labels her mother's actions as "aggressive."

the conflicts that she and her daughter, Mary, experienced. In Mary's second visit to the clinic, we explored in greater detail Mrs. Smith's hitting, shoving, scratching, and pushing episodes. Table 5.1 shows an updated functional analysis table that was the result of this discussion.

As seen in Table 5.1, it turned out that Mrs. Smith's physically "aggressive" behaviors toward Mary always occurred in the context of bowel and urinary continence care. By using an A • B • C functional analytic approach in this way, Mary was able to see the connection between Mrs. Smith's seemingly aggressive behavior and Mary's approach to assistive continence care. Mary then realized that she was treating her mother much like she used to treat her now teenage son when he was a toddler years ago. Mary decided to hire a home health assistant for Mrs. Smith's personal care. Mrs. Smith did not object to help provided by a nonfamily member, who was able to assist her in a professional, respectful, and matter-of-fact way, and Mary was greatly relieved, freed from the primary responsibility for this difficult aspect of care. Once this particularly strong context for conflict between the two of them was removed, Mrs. Smith completely stopped physically affronting her daughter.

2. Ruling Out Sensory Loss

Although degenerative dementia leads to a progressive decline in a person's ability to communicate, one of the prime features of being human is our continuing wish to connect with others, particularly via the written and spoken word. Achieving this connection becomes even more effortful when a person with dementia cannot hear or see accurately. Loss of vision and hearing makes it difficult to engage in many meaningful life activities, both large and small: watching a movie with your spouse, seeing your grandchild graduate, talking about an article you read in the morning newspaper over coffee. Sensory loss also deprives the person with dementia of access to the nonverbal, verbal, and tonal cues we all use to interpret and respond to social situations. Especially when dementia is only mild, it is difficult to tell sensory and cognitive losses apart. Does the person have hearing loss, or does he or she not understand the meaning of what was said? Is he or she not able to feed himself or herself, or can she not see the white food on his or her white plate?

Because of the inability of individuals with dementia to describe their internal experiences, the diagnosis of sensory loss can be difficult. Most people with dementia do not realize that they would benefit from glasses or a hearing aid, that their prescription is outdated and new devices are in order, or in a more dramatic case, that their hearing aid batteries have gone dead. It is not uncommon to meet people in residential care or skilled nursing homes without their glasses or hearing aids, lost once upon a time and never replaced. To determine need, you can ask for and check photos of the person for prosthetic devices. In addition, observation of the person is invaluable. Do you see any behaviors that would be indicative of hearing loss? Age-related hearing loss tends to affect higher frequency tones; does the person become more engaged when you deepen your voice without making it louder? Is the person speaking loudly or increasing the volume of the radio or television? Is he coming close to hear you, or does he cup his ear? Is he watching your face and lips intently? Likewise, do your observations indicate that visual loss may be present? Has the person stopped participating in meaningful activities that require visual acuity? Does he have trouble grasping or pouring? Has she given up reading? Does she have difficulty finding items that are right in front of her? Do his eyes look strained, red, or teary? Does he seem to walk more carefully? If you or the caregiver suspects a sensory deficit, then a referral to a specialist is in order. Ophthalmologists; optometrists; audiologists; ear, nose, and, throat specialists; and others will help determine whether and to what degree sensory loss and sensory barriers to communication are present.

Using Prosthetic Devices

When you assess for sensory loss, you may hear from caregivers that they took Dad to the audiologist a decade ago and purchased expensive hearing aids that Dad never wore. Here, a functional A • B • C assessment as to what interferes with using the prescribed prosthetics is helpful. Engaging with others is usually a pretty powerful motivator, but there are a variety of reasons that a person will reject the assistive devices that would reduce their social isolation. These include the following: (a) The person does not know he or she needs prosthetics; (b) using the prosthetic involves an intricate or uncomfortable process, such as inserting or adjusting hearing aids, that the person has not mastered; (c) the prosthetics do not work correctly or do not meet the needs of the person, as when hearing aids amplify background noise rather than human speech, or trifocals require adjusting to too many corrective visual ranges; or (d) the client's social environment is too demanding, and sensory loss provides an "exit with dignity" from overwhelming visual or auditory stimulation. Again, detective work is needed, and the solutions and necessary compromises that will work best will vary with each person.

Case Example of Sensory Loss: Follow-Up With Mrs. Flynn

When Mrs. Flynn was seen in our clinic, she was alert, friendly, and cooperative. Her MMSE score was 18/30. She easily engaged in conversation with the treating clinician. However, she was not able to explain the reason she was being seen in the clinic and did not indicate that she remembered having any problems paying her bills. She talked repeatedly about what a handsome man and good dancer her deceased husband was and about her darling cockatiel, Smokey. She readily agreed to any follow-up visits at her home, despite the fact that she did not seem to understand their purpose. Because Mrs. Flynn seemed unable to orient to current context or to provide informed consent for our services, Elder Protective Services initiated guardianship proceedings, and a public guardian was appointed 3 months later.

Shortly thereafter, Mrs. Flynn's guardian contacted us to say that Mrs. Flynn had been admitted to a hospital emergency room. Neighbors had notified the guardian after observing Mrs. Flynn moving knickknacks and wall hangings out of her house. The guardian said that Mrs. Flynn "did not make any sense" and could not be persuaded to interrupt her moving endeavor. When the support center clinician arrived at the emergency room, Mrs. Flynn was fully clothed, lying on a bed. She was confused and did not interact appropriately with anyone who spoke to her. The emergency room physician diagnosed acute delirium. The clinician suggested to the physician to check the functionality of Mrs. Flynn's hearing aids. When a nurse's aide asked for permission to remove the hearing aids, Mrs. Flynn did not respond. She turned her head appropriately on physical prompting, yet looked bewildered. The nurse's aide found that both hearing aid batteries were dead. After the batteries were changed, Mrs. Flynn began orienting to people and within 20 min asked to return home. To the nurse's aide, who did not have much dementia care experience, the recovery seemed "magical." The guardian was alerted to prompt Mrs. Flynn and, if necessary, assist her in replacing her hearing aid batteries on a regular basis.

3. Ruling Out Adverse Medication Effects

When a person ages, the way her body absorbs, distributes, and eliminates medication changes. More than any other age group, older adults are at high risk of adverse events resulting from the medication they take. This high risk is due to multiple factors, including polypharmacy and unforeseen or unstudied drug interactions, lack of client adherence to an often complex medication regimen, lack of medication-side-effects monitoring, inappropriate prescribing for older adults, and idiosyncratic drug–body interactions. Indeed, adverse events are so common among older persons that it has been said that "any new symptom in an older patient should be considered a possible drug effect until proven otherwise" (Avorn & Wang, 2005, p. 36). A layperson would expect adverse events to occur after there have been changes to the medication regimen. However, the long-term properties of drugs combined with age-related physiological changes can also lead to adverse effects even when a medication has been taken for years. Thus, rather than asking, "Has there been a recent medication change?" the question should be, "What factors within the medication regimen could potentially cause these complaints or behavioral changes?" This question is best asked of a pharmacist who is certified in geriatrics. Geriatric pharmacists study pharmacokinetics, pharmacodynamics, and biotransformation specific to older adults and may be able to predict or identify adverse events in your older client on the basis of his or her unique medical and health profile. Your role will be to collaborate with the caregiver in compiling and communicating essential information about affective, behavioral, and cognitive changes, without which the pharmacist would be unable to detect potential adverse effects.

Adverse Medication Effects in Persons With Dementia

Most of your clients with dementia will be older adults, so all of the medication-related risks mentioned earlier will apply to them. However, there are additional adverse effects risks associated with medication use in persons with dementia that are important for you to know:

- Adults with dementia are generally excluded from clinical trials in which medications have been tested (if they have been tested on geriatric populations at all). Neurodegenerative changes in the brain caused by a dementing illness may result in dramatically different treatment responses to medications than those found in normal older adults. For example, most individuals with dementia of the Lewy body type are unable to tolerate typical or atypical antipsychotics, and in extreme cases, use of these medications can even cause death in these patients.

- As verbal reasoning ability decreases, individuals with dementia may not be able to "talk themselves through" the side effects of a drug. For example, a prescribing physician may say, "These eye drops may sting or burn a little bit when you put them in, but they will keep your glaucoma from progressing." For individuals with dementia who are unable to remember these instructions or understand the purpose of the medication, the eye drops are simply intolerable. The person with dementia will react negatively every time the caregiver approaches to administer the drops. If a pill is hard to swallow, people with dementia may spit it out. If it leaves an unpleasant taste in their mouth, they may accuse their caregiver of poisoning their food. If they have never taken medications in the past, they may refuse them outright now. Struggles over medication delivery can greatly compromise the caregiver–care recipient relationship.
- It bears repeating that most individuals with dementia are unable to reliably report internal events and so may not be able to tell us how drugs are affecting them. Most medications carry a long list of possible side effects, some of which are rare but quite severe in their health implications. Physicians rely on timely patient self-reports to know when medication side effects occur. Proxy monitoring by caregivers of affect, cognition, and behavior is crucial to detecting adverse medication effects, but even then, important symptoms can be missed. You should encourage caregivers to be proactive with their doctors to ensure that care recipients are prescribed medications with the lowest risk profiles to minimize the danger of unreported effects.
- Individuals with dementia may not receive proper interventions for adverse events because these side effects may be incorrectly attributed to the degenerative dementia itself. Many drugs, regardless of whether they were intended to affect mood and behavior, do produce inadvertent mood and behavior changes. An older adult may react to the drug with increased confusion (e.g., digoxin, antihistamines), agitation (e.g., bronchodilators), or hallucinations or psychosis (e.g., levodopa, procainamide, corticosteroids). When a person already has a dementia diagnosis, it may be presumed that the increased confusion, agitation, or hallucinations are a result of progressing disease rather than a medication adverse event. You, as the client's advocate, can facilitate properly ruling out medication effects by ensuring that the treating physician and geriatric pharmacist have a detailed list of all prescription medication and detailed infor-

mation about observed affective, cognitive, and behavioral changes.

- Last, lack of medication regimen adherence puts persons with dementia at a particular risk of adverse effects. Individuals such as Mrs. Flynn who live alone may manage their own medications haphazardly because of their memory and comprehension problems. Alternatively, well-meaning caregivers may not follow doctors' orders but administer medications depending on whether their loved one has a "good" or a "bad" day. They may add over-the-counter medications or nutraceuticals that are described as curative on Internet discussion boards. They may even administer their own medications to the care recipient on an "as-needed" basis. Some caregivers also omit medications the care recipient refuses to take (e.g., the care recipient will only take red pills and refuse yellow ones). For all these reasons, we recommend that your evaluation always include a thorough examination of medication management practices. If there is evidence of medication nonadherence, a functional A • B • C assessment is useful. What are possible barriers (activators) to following doctor's orders? What does nonadherence accomplish for the caregiver or care recipient (consequences)? After you have obtained a detailed description of all the contextual factors involved in the nonadherence behavior, you can start a collaborative problem-solving process.

Medications "for" Dementia

Many family caregivers are under the impression that cognitive function enhancing or psychotropic medications prescribed for the affective and behavioral changes in dementia are curative. One of your roles is to educate caregivers about the role medication plays in dementia care and to make sure they understand the risks and benefits and are giving truly informed consent for their use.[2] We find that many families run through the gamut of prescriptions, only to become discouraged when "nothing is helping" and their loved ones do not regain their cognitive abilities. Education includes awareness that so-called cognitive function–enhancing

---

[2]For example, the cognitive function–enhancing medications commonly used for the treatment of Alzheimer's disease can produce cholinergic effects, including urinary incontinence and diarrhea (Gill et al., 2005). Advocacy involves alerting caregivers to the prescription information and potential side effects of these and other medications so that these symptoms are not mistakenly diagnosed as dementia-related and unnecessarily treated.

drugs may slow the progression of dementia in some cases but not all, that they are not designed to be curative, and that we cannot predict in advance who will benefit and who will not. Clients should be informed that prescriptions for affective and behavioral disturbances in dementia are currently an off-label use; as of December 2009, there were no drugs approved by the U.S. Food and Drug Administration for the treatment of behavioral disturbances in dementia.[3] Because evidence-based nonpharmacological interventions for many symptoms are available, these should always be considered the first line of treatment.

It is essential for families of persons with dementia to collaborate with medical professionals to enhance their loved ones' quality of care. When educating families, we are careful to point out the complexities of dementia care and the challenge physicians face when managing illnesses in persons who are unable to self-report. It is crucial that families understand their pivotal advocacy role, which is based on their close knowledge of the person with dementia. Our goal is to train caregivers to provide important information about their loved one's functioning in a timely fashion, even when they traditionally might have assumed that "doctor knows best" and avoided sharing necessary information with an authority figure.

Case Example of Adverse Medication Effects: Mrs. Smith

Before coming to our clinic, Mrs. Smith had been institutionalized several times for agitated behavioral outbursts and resistance to care. At the time of her referral to our outpatient clinic, her medication list included five psychotropic medications prescribed to alter affect and behavior (one antidepressant, one antiseizure medication, two antipsychotics, one anxiolytic) and two cognitive function enhancers. We informed the geriatric pharmacist that bowel and urinary incontinence as well as accusatory behavior continued to be problems. A medication review suggested that a common side effect of the antidepressant was a distorted or "metallic" taste and that the incontinence could be caused by one of the cognitive enhancers. The medication review also proposed discontinuing one of the atypical antipsychotics. After Mrs. Smith's psychiatrist implemented the recommended changes, Mary reported that Mrs. Smith's accusations of being poisoned stopped. In addition, Mary's incontinence "accidents" completely ceased.

---

[3]Not only is there limited evidence supporting the effectiveness of psychotropic medication use for cognitively impaired individuals but also atypical and typical antipsychotic medications have been linked to increased mortality of individuals with dementia due to cerebrovascular events ("Antipsychotic drugs for dementia," 2009; Ballard et al., 2009; Meeks & Jeste, 2008; U.S. Food and Drug Administration, 2009a, 2009b).

4. Ruling Out Medical Illnesses

It is important to rule out medication side effects for changes in dementia because the majority of our clients have multiple chronic illnesses for which they are taking medications. A dementia diagnosis is not protective against concurrent diagnoses of hypertension, Type 2 diabetes, cardiovascular disease, and osteoporosis, to name only a few of the most common age-related conditions. Many of these illnesses must be carefully managed not only to avoid unnecessarily compromised physical debility but also to reduce risk of further accelerated cognitive and functional decline. There is increasing evidence that lowering cholesterol and blood pressure levels, controlling or preventing diabetes, and maintaining a healthy body mass index are as important for reducing the risk of developing Alzheimer's disease as they are for protecting against heart disease, stroke, and cancer. It is less clear to what extent appropriate management of chronic illnesses slows cognitive decline in persons with existing dementia diagnoses, but it is safe to say that what is healthy for the heart is healthy for the brain, and those with already compromised brain function should do whatever possible to preserve those brain cells that are still intact.

Managing acute and chronic medical illness is also incredibly important for the goal of reducing functional excess disability for persons with dementia. At the start of this chapter we talked about the impact on mood and function that we all experience when we are feeling sick, tired, or uncomfortable, and that is only magnified in persons with dementia. Infections, including urinary tract infections, pneumonia, skin infections, sepsis, and diarrhea are not only common causes of delirium and other acute changes in behavior but also a frequent cause of death of those with severe dementia (Kukull et al., 1994). Cognitively impaired individuals are more prone to fatigue, perhaps because they work harder to cope with all aspects of daily living. Fatigue has been identified as an important component of the cyclic "sundowning" agitation some persons with dementia exhibit. Another particularly important activator for many behavior problems in persons with dementia is pain. Have you ever tried sitting all day? People with advanced dementia who are confined to wheelchairs may experience bodily aches and pain beyond our imagination. Increased inactivity and immobility leads to stiffness and muscle atrophy that makes ambulation and self-care activities painful and exhausting. It is not surprising that sores emerge from pressure, shearing forces, moisture (e.g., from incontinence), and friction. Some studies of long-term care facilities report that among individuals identified to be at risk of pressure ulcers, up to 47% had or developed such ulcers during a 3-month period (Horn et al., 2002). Even for ambulatory individuals, pain can develop and go unrecognized for prolonged periods if the person with dementia is unable to locate the pain site or describe what they are feeling. To illustrate this important issue, consider the following case.

Case 3. Mrs. Puttani: Helping Severely Impaired Individuals in Skilled Nursing Facilities

Mrs. Dotson contacts you and says she needs help with her mother, 93-year-old Mrs. Puttani, who has lived in a skilled nursing facility for the past 2 years. Mrs. Puttani has diagnoses of moderate to severe vascular dementia and macular degeneration, and she is wheelchair-bound since she broke her hip some years ago. According to Mrs. Dotson, Mrs. Puttani hardly speaks anymore. Mrs. Dotson is concerned because staff members have reported that Mrs. Puttani has become "mean" and has tried to hit or scratch staff members at the nursing facility. Mrs. Dotson is at a loss. She says that her mother used to be a schoolteacher, a veritable "Ms. Manners," and that her mother's behavior is out of character. She states that the attending physician told her that her mother's behaviors are an inevitable consequence of the disease.

Mrs. Dotson, who is her mother's attorney-in-fact, arranges for you to obtain a release for an exchange of information with the nursing facility and its medical director. When you meet Mrs. Puttani, she is sitting in her wheelchair at a lunch table with other residents who are not able to feed themselves. Mrs. Puttani listens to your introduction, and nods. You notice that she is not able to take verbal turns with you in conversation, but she engages in nonverbal behavior (nodding) and inserts sentences here and there. She has an MMSE score of 2, seems restless and talks about "going away." Her severe word-finding difficulties result in metaphorical or circumlocutory speech, yet she still seems intent on participating. For example, she repeatedly compliments you by saying, "You have such nice teeth," which seems to be a comment on your smile and friendliness. You notice that Mrs. Puttani's face is a bit contorted, as if in pain. She does not smile, and she sometimes frowns. When you ask the certified nursing assistant, she states that Mrs. Puttani "always looks angry."

In preparation for a meeting with nursing home staff and administration to talk about Mrs. Puttani, it would be helpful to briefly review the principles we have been developing throughout this book as they might apply to this case.

- D: Discuss concerns respectfully. What do staff members mean when they say that Mrs. Puttani has become "mean"? Does she exhibit other problem behaviors besides those that the daughter has described to you? What circumstances and stressors of their job may be affecting Mrs. Puttani's care? Do they feel that they have enough time to help all the residents as they would like, or are they shorthanded and frequently rushed? What kinds of dementia education training programs have they received?

- A: Ameliorate excess disability. Has Mrs. Puttani developed any new medical illness that the daughter did not mention? Has her change in behavior occurred suddenly or gradually over time? What kinds of physical rehabilitation or pain management does she routinely receive for her broken hip? How has her macular degeneration progressed since admission to the nursing facility?
- N: Nurture the dyad. What is Mrs. Puttani's typical day like? Is she regularly engaged in activities at the facility that are enjoyable to her and appropriate for her level of function? How often is her daughter able to visit, and what do they do when she comes?
- C: Create contextual solutions. What exactly is happening when Mrs. Puttani gets upset? Is there any pattern to when it happens (e.g., time of day), where it happens (e.g., dining room, hallway, her bedroom, shower), or who is around (e.g., particular staff, other residents)? How do staff members respond? Do their responses make the situation better or worse?
- E: Enjoy the journey. What can Mrs. Puttani's daughter tell you and the staff that would help you know and understand her better? Do workers at the nursing facility like Mrs. Puttani? Does she have friends at the facility, and if so, who are they, and how often do they spend time with her?

After meeting with Mrs. Puttani and her daughter, you interview the staff members who allege attacks by Mrs. Puttani. They tell you that until recently they had a good relationship with her. Your queries about possible activators and consequences for her behaviors yield the information organized in an A • B • C format in Table 5.2.

TABLE 5.2
Overview of Steps in the A • B • Cs for Mrs. Puttani

Activators	Mrs. Puttani's behaviors	Consequences
Staff members tell Mrs. Puttani to stop what she is doing. Staff members stop Mrs. Puttani's wheelchair in the hallway. Staff members prevent Mrs. Puttani from entering another resident's room.	Hitting, shoving, pushing, yelling at staff	Staff members reason with Mrs. Puttani. Staff members show frustrated and angry behavior toward Mrs. Puttani. Staff members let Mrs. Puttani continue on her way.

Further investigation revealed that these incidences were novel; up until the past week they had not occurred at all, and now they were happening several times a day. A record review showed that in addition to severe visual loss and dementia, Mrs. Puttani had a history of urinary tract infections. The last urinary analysis had been performed 5 weeks previously. Following our conversation with Mrs. Puttani's charge nurse, her physician ordered new labs, and a urinary tract infection was confirmed. We may speculate that Mrs. Puttani was in pain, trying to return to her room or attempting to find a bathroom when staff members blocked her way. Although staff behavior was the proximal activator for Mrs. Puttani's responses, the urinary tract infection was the distal or ultimate cause of her behavior. As is typical with the management of pain-related conditions, on treatment of the urinary tract infection Mrs. Puttani's out-of-character behaviors disappeared. Staff members were informed that the disruptive behavior had been Mrs. Puttani's way of letting them know something was wrong; the care staff's relationship with Mrs. Puttani returned to being friendly and affectionate.

Unfortunately, Mrs. Puttani's case is no isolated incident. Providing adequate pain management is one of the greatest challenges of dementia care, but when pain is managed, disruptive behaviors may disappear, as in Mrs. Puttani's example. Thus, it is up to caregivers to watch behavior carefully and be vigilant for any change or unusual occurrence. Our clients' behavior says what words cannot.

Dental Pain in Persons With Dementia

One often overlooked source of pain and discomfort can be found within your client's mouth. In our experience, many clients have gone for years without dental checkups and may suffer from teeth decay, toothaches, sore and infected gums, or have broken partials or dentures. Collaboration with social workers may be necessary to identify professionals qualified to provide proper dental care to cognitively impaired individuals.

In addition, your participation in exploring treatment options with family members may be essential. When a client's dental condition is severe enough to warrant teeth extraction and dentures, new obstacles can present themselves. Does the client remember having had dental surgery? Does he or she have postsurgical pain or increased confusion from pain medications? Is the client able to understand the purpose of dentures? Clients will need assistance inserting the dentures in the morning (using verbal or physical prompts or modeling if somebody else with dentures can be found), removing them for nightly cleaning, and monitoring their proper fit over time. This routine does not always go smoothly. For some clients with dementia, losing one's teeth is shocking. We have seen severely impaired individuals who were terrified by the feel and the look of their toothless gums. In extreme cases, having a mouth suddenly emptied of one's teeth is like suddenly having a limb removed, and it can trigger fear and distress every time the dentures are taken out. Thus, before embarking onto the journey of oral surgery and dentures with a person with severe cognitive impairment, it is important to explore all alternatives, their risks and benefits, and the possible complications that can arise from the prolonged recovery and adjustment period.

5. Ruling Out Depression

The last major comorbid condition to consider ruling out when clients exhibit changes in mood and behavior is depression. Withdrawal from activities is typical when a person is diagnosed with a degenerative cognitive impairment. Dementia-related changes in executive functioning can produce declines in motivation and ability to initiate activity. However, withdrawal from pleasurable activities can also be a both a symptom and cause of depression. If you use the A • B • C contingency table to think about how your client's activities have changed, you will often see that activities that were highly rewarding in the past are now being avoided because they are occasions for feelings of failure and social discomfort. For example, recall the simplified chain of events described in Chapter 2 with the professor who developed word-finding difficulties. Her increasing problems with public speaking (B) led to a decrease in attendance at her lectures (C). This decrease in attendance at lectures (A) caused the professor to decline future speaking engagements (B). Because being a successful public speaker was a source of pleasure and an important role identity, as her speaking engagements declined, the professor began to feel cut off from her professional colleagues, disappointed in herself, or even useless (C). This could then lead to further withdrawal and social isolation and feelings of boredom, sadness, and loss, deepening the professor's cycle into depression.

The best general antidote to depressed behavioral patterns is continued or increased engagement in pleasant and personally meaningful activities. Because of the importance for both caregivers and care recipients of maintaining involvement in activities that bring a sense of joy and purpose to life, we talk much more about this in subsequent chapters of this book.

Detecting Health Status Changes of Concern

It is interesting that high frequency meaningful or "index" activities can actually help us detect comorbid medical conditions or adverse effects in cognitively impaired populations. When clients suddenly lose interest in valued activities, it is important to rule out illnesses, medication effects, or other adverse events (Reiss & Aman, 1998). Hanan, for example, was an octogenarian with vascular dementia, hypertension, renal failure, and Type 2 diabetes, living in a skilled nursing facility. Her high-frequency activities at the facility included attendance at meals in the dining hall, greeting and making small talk with visitors, and "reading" books. Although she did not understand what she had read, she would turn the pages of her paperback novels, just like she had done in the past, and mark each book with a small penciled x on the inside of the cover page once she was done with it. Monitoring of Hanan's high-frequency activities was a good indicator of how she felt. If she declined visitors or sent them away, trouble was brewing; over the course of her years in the nursing home, she had had pneumonia, several urinary tract infections, and a beginning pressure sore that had been detected by changes in her regular activities. If she missed breakfast, the nurses knew that Hanan had been too dizzy to get up, and they would work with her primary care physician and urologist to monitor her glucose and blood pressure levels and adjust her medications as required. Toward the end of Hanan's life, she stopped "reading" altogether; at that point, it was time for a hospice assessment.

Establishing Collaborations

Throughout this chapter we have talked about ruling out a variety of comorbid conditions that can increase client excess disability. Ruling out virtually all of these requires close collaboration between caregivers and any number of health care providers, including physicians, geriatric pharmacists, nurses, and a variety of allied health and behavioral health specialists. Are medical specialists involved in your client's care? What about psychiatrists? Is your client in a long-term care facility that is mandated to undergo monthly medication review? Does he or she have a primary care physician? Is the family in agreement with the health care recommendations that have been made? Is a caregiver available to monitor ongoing treatment adherence? Does the caregiver know what to do and who to call if something goes wrong? No matter what your professional background, it is your task to ensure that a collaborative system of health care provision is in effect for your cognitively impaired client.

Collaborating With Other Professionals

The ideal, but rare, situation is one in which a primary care physician has known a patient for decades and you can work with this physician to establish a system of care. In this case, when the patient develops dementia, the primary care physician has a baseline of social interactions with the patient and will automatically take steps to rule out possible comorbid conditions that may be causing observed changes. Regrettably, many people do not have an established primary care physician. If they do, a move to long-term care usually prevents continuity of care because most physicians do not offer services in facilities. As a general rule, the less a health care provider knows the person with dementia, the more important is the provision of background and baseline information to facilitate the detection of adverse events and to prevent their attribution to the dementing disease.

Our approach to working with other professionals assumes that we all agree that optimizing a person's care is highly valued, that need is high, and that time is in short supply. If possible, we limit our contact with other professionals to brief, bulleted faxes, detailing caregivers' observations of behavior and affect and asking for medical clearance or for specific conditions to be ruled out before implementing behavioral health care interventions. We include the necessary releases for the exchange of medical information in our correspondence, even if we have sent them before, and ask for a brief update when results are in. When working with clients in residential care settings, we might ask for face-to-face meetings with facility staff who can then initiate the ruling out of necessary conditions.

Our experience has been that when comorbidities are suspected and ruled out, leading to improvements in clients' functioning, community health care providers become more likely to routinely assess for contributing comorbidities in the future. The emergency room physician and nurse who witnessed the dissolution of Mrs. Flynn's delirium-like condition will be more likely to check for hearing-aid functioning when the next patient comes through the door. The nurse in Mrs. Puttani's facility will be more likely to run a urinalysis immediately. The client's recovery reinforces the health care providers' behavior. Thus, you have the opportunity to set a system of "checks and rule-outs" into motion. Opportunity, as Thomas Edison famously remarked, is missed by most people because it comes dressed in overalls and looks like work. By doing the work of helping our professional colleagues look for comorbid contributions to behavior changes in cognitively impaired individuals, we may reap the long-term rewards of seeing the prevention of excess disability become the expected practice in community care.

Collaborating With the Caregiving Dyad

When providing quality health care to persons with dementia, all roads lead to the primary caregiver(s) who see the care recipient frequently, if not every day. As with every other aspect of dementia care, the best-designed health management plan will fail if the person with dementia is unable to remember what to do or to report problems that may arise. Thus, collaboration with caregivers is an essential component of reducing excess disability in our cognitively impaired clients. Caregivers often need coaching to organize a care recipient's complex health care appointments and treatment, and you can be an invaluable ally in this process. Caregivers also need guidelines for recognizing behavioral changes that may indicate the presence of a comorbid condition or medication side effect, so that an appropriate health care professional can be contacted and the care recipient can be treated as promptly as possible. In our experience, there is nothing more fulfilling than a caregiver reporting a successful and independent resolution of an adverse event-related problem. Last, caregivers often need assistance dealing with care recipients' refusal to follow treatment recommendations. An A • B • C functional analysis can help caregivers identify possible activators for the care recipient's behavior and whether their own communication style and response is making the situation better or worse. However, some problematic caregiver–care recipient interactions around medical treatment are grounded in deeper and older stressors in the relationship that have been exacerbated by the presence of the dementing illness. In the next chapter, we introduce our final case, that of Mr. Malloy, to talk about how to nurture and strengthen the dyadic relationship as a way of ultimately strengthening the entire collaborative community of care.

6

NURTURE THE DYAD: STRENGTHENING CAREGIVER PARTNERSHIPS

As is evident in Chapter 5, effective dementia care is a collaborative effort: No single individual with dementia, no single caregiver, and no single professional is able to go the distance alone and without support. For this reason, one of the primary goals of treatment is to generate a community of care. The relationships between the person with dementia and his or her loved ones are at the heart of this community. The preserving, restoring, or strengthening of these relationships is one of the most rewarding aspects of behavioral health care practice.

RELATIONSHIPS FROM A CONTEXTUAL POINT OF VIEW

There is a concept used in couples therapy called *reinforcement erosion* (Jacobson & Margolin, 1979) that can be useful in understanding the process of how relationships change when one person in the dyad develops dementia. When two people initially fall in love, they respond to almost everything the other person says and does with positive attention, smiling, nodding, and an array of romantic gestures. However, with time, repetition, and the burdens of the daily grind, words and actions that were once intriguing or endearing lose their magic and become stale. As a result, relationships experience a slowly creeping decrease in the frequency with which the partners' behaviors are acknowledged and reinforced. They may start complaining about "being taken for granted," and yet feel unable to put their finger on exactly what is the matter. In the language of the contextual model outlined in Chapter 2, *extinction* is occurring. The partners are inadvertently withdrawing those patterns of responding that used to maintain the still desired romantic connection. It is worthwhile noting that all close relationships, whether spousal, parent–child, extended family, or community friendships, are vulnerable to this same gradual, almost unnoticeable drift in intimacy over time. Successful relationships intentionally create opportunities to counteract this drift with planned romantic vacations, weekend getaways, neighborhood gatherings, family sit-down meals, office retreats, holiday celebrations, letters and calls, or even simple breaks in busy lives to listen to one another and maintain the valued personal connection.

HOW DEMENTIA CHANGES RELATIONSHIPS

Progressive degenerative dementia shifts this gradual, barely detectable decline in intimacy to a punctuated, clearly discernible jolt. Even when dementia is mild, relationships start to change because the partners suddenly are no longer behaving as expected. Caregivers make everyday, familiar requests or statements (e.g., "Could you look at what's going on with the water heater, please?" "When's dinner ready?" "What's on TV?" "Have you paid the cable bill?"), and the care recipient responds with an inappropriate comment or action or says and does nothing at all. From the point of view of the person with dementia, his response makes sense and is the best he can muster. For the wife who comes downstairs to check on the water heater and finds the basement flooded and her husband happily tinkering in his shop a few yards away, the situation is incomprehensible. Caregivers' smiling, nodding, and affectionate tones of voice are replaced by bewilderment, frowning, complaining, and nagging. A spouse or child may ask for explanations that the person with dementia is unable to render: "Why did you comment on Fran's weight gain?" "Why did you change your mind about attending the social?" "Why didn't you tell me the bill had not been paid?" "Why didn't you meet me at the time we agreed?" The person with dementia does not understand why suddenly everything he does is being questioned and criticized and in turn reacts defensively. Reversing this cascading collapse in relationship requires helping the caregiver and care recipient recognize what is happening. If we can normalize the emotional turmoil that both persons are experiencing and help caregivers shift their expectations for both the care recipient and themselves, it becomes possible for the dyad to build a resilient foundation for all the relationship changes that are yet to come.

REEXAMINING EXPECTATIONS

If we are to help caregivers and care recipients preserve and strengthen relationships, we have to first assist them to see that dementia is changing the (often unspoken) "rules" that have been operating for years. In Chapter 2, we laid out the principles of reinforcement and extinction that, as described earlier, are part of the ebb and flow in all relationships. In addition, in the same chapter, we talked about the importance of social beliefs and values in the development and maintenance of human behavior. Caregivers and care recipients, like all of us, have grown up with certain familial, social or religious, and cultural expectations of how people should behave in certain situations. For example, in many Asian cultures, there is a strong emphasis on filial piety, which emphasizes respecting one's parents, not bringing dishonor to one's family, and taking care of one's parents. Failure to do so brings shame on both the parent and child. The adult son from such a culture is thus placed in a difficult bind when his father with dementia takes steps to sell the family business to invest in a pyramid scheme. To directly challenge his father would be inconceivable. To do nothing would mean that his parents' retirement security could be destroyed. Reasoning respectfully with his father has proved ineffectual. The frustration and anger the son feels toward the older man may feel shocking and disgraceful. Is there any way to assist the son in this situation?

One way caregivers can get "unstuck" when they are caught in such a dilemma is to consider whether their expectations for the care recipient are still reasonable with regard to the specific problem situation. In the example, reviewing details of the father's plans and actions to date would likely provide multiple examples of his memory loss; recent problems with attention and concentration, reasoning, and judgment; and uncharacteristic mood swings. Considering these examples together would clarify which aspects of the family financial planning and control should no longer be exclusively in the father's hands. It is critical here for the son to understand that the father's deficits in this specific area in no way make him less worthy of filial respect. They also do not mean that none of the father's business opinions should be considered or that the father should not retain control over other aspects of family life. Helping the son understand that there is a specific dementia-related reason for him to intervene in this specific situation can break down the impasse to action. The son may realize that by quietly assuming financial authority for the family business he is actually protecting his father's honor, which would be threatened if they were to be left penniless. If he can grasp that his father's cognitive changes make him unable to fully appreciate the consequences of his behavior, then the son will be more patient and feel less shame when his father becomes angry with him. In this case, by doing what was previously unthinkable—unobtrusively taking over management of the family finances despite his father's wishes to continue in that role—the son paradoxically is honoring and respecting the older man.

We see in this example that as events unfold, successful caregivers shift their own self-expectations as well as their expectations of the care recipient. In the beginning, the son would have rejected any action that could be viewed as deceptive or defiant of his father's wishes, because he wanted to be a good son. What changed was not the son's value system; being a good son remained of greatest importance to him. What changed was his understanding of how to best practice or live out his values. Changes in family roles and expectations about what one is capable of or allowed to do are part and parcel of being a resilient dementia caregiver. Husbands take over housekeeping chores that were previously "women's work" and discover that they like to bake. Wives who never balanced a checkbook find they have a knack for picking good investments and driving a hard bargain at the car dealership. A previously shy and soft-spoken daughter becomes an assertive health care advocate for her declining parents. However, these changes come gradually and can be accompanied by considerable angst along the way, particularly if the care recipient does not understand or like the new ordering of things.

Parent–child shifts in role relationships are often the most difficult of all because the expectations on both sides are deeply entrenched. It can be helpful for caregivers to think through what makes their own role changes so difficult to accept. It almost always turns out that the difficulty lies in the fact that either (a) the caregiver and/or care recipient are not living up to some ideal standard (i.e., what a good husband/wife/parent/child "should" do or act like) or (b) the caregiver's life has become so different from what was anticipated and planned that the caregiver feels completely out of control. In the latter situation, thinking about expectations and values may not suggest a way forward. Rather the caregiver needs to try something completely different. We suggest that what they need to do is give up the struggle.

SETTING A NEW CONTEXT FOR CARE

It is common for caregivers in the midst of crisis to believe that the "the problem" that needs fixing is the apparently improper or unreasonable actions of the person with dementia. Hence, the solution to the problem is that the unreasonable behavior simply needs to be stopped. Most caregiving dyads have a history of solving problems together, and so when difficulties first arise, caregivers try the familiar strategies that have served them in the past. These past and familiar strategies usually involve some combination of talking, questioning, reasoning, coming to some shared agreement, confronting, arguing, threatening, acquiescing, apologizing, or ignoring the problem in the hope that it will go away. Of course, because the dementia is progressive, it usually does not go away, and the whole problem-solving cycle begins anew. The man whose formerly thrifty wife is now maxing out her credit cards buying extravagant gifts is loathe to cancel her cards or take them away, but he is also infuriated when she continues to spend so much money after promising the week before to stop. In cases where the care recipient does not yet have a dementia diagnosis or the cognitive and functional impairment are relatively mild, spouses and children can struggle in this unproductive problem-solving cycle for years. Many caregivers we encounter are exhausted and describe feeling stuck, hopeless, frustrated, and discouraged because nothing they do seems to help.

Surprisingly, what caregivers actually need to do in this situation is give up the problem-solving strategies that worked before and are so ineffective now. We tell caregivers that their situation is like being in a tug-of-war where the caregiver is holding one end of a rope and a terrible monster is standing across a dreadful abyss holding the other end.[1] Each time the caregivers pull hard and gain an inch of separation from the abyss (e.g., get the care-recipient to cease a problematic behavior with verbal reasoning), the dementia monster pulls even harder and undoes the tiny gain. For example, consider the caregiver who has a reasonable discussion with her care recipient husband who is emptying his dresser drawers and scattering the contents all over the bedroom. The husband apologizes for making a mess and the caregiver feels hopeful and satisfied. An hour later she finds him searching for something in his closet. When she asks, "What do you need?" her husband replies, "I need you to fill my prescription for t-shirts, 'cause I'm running out of them." How does the caregiver feel now? Her earlier thoughts that things are not really so bad as the doctors say "fight" with feelings of devastation and fear. As time passes, some caregivers spend a lot of time and effort in the struggle to hold fearful, angry, or judgmental thoughts and feelings at bay. They may cling to old ways of doing things to avoid the implications of the need to change their behavior. Resisting change is tantamount to clutching the rope.

---

[1]This metaphor is one commonly used in acceptance and commitment therapy (ACT), a contextual form of therapy developed by Dr. Steven C. Hayes in Reno. Readers interested in finding out more specifics about ACT, including its underlying philosophy of science and foundation in behavior analysis, are encouraged to read Hayes, Strosahl, and Wilson (1999). Reviews of empirical studies to date using ACT as a therapeutic modality can be found in Hayes, Luoma, Bond, Masuda, and Lillis (2006) and Hayes, Masuda, Bissett, Luoma, and Guerrero (2004). Adaptations of ACT particular to anxiety (Eifert & Forsyth, 2005), depression (Zettle, 2007), and couples therapy (Harris, 2009) are available.

In our work with family caregivers, we try to help them to see that giving up the struggle and accepting the reality of a spouse or parent's progressive decline and the unpredictability and mixed emotions this creates does not mean there is nothing to do and no hope for things getting better. It simply means recognizing that the rules of engagement have changed. Powerful expectations of how things "should be" or "used to be" in the imagined future or the remembered past trap caregivers in this tug-of-war. Caregivers may feel that altering these expectations—and changing one's behavior to provide a more prosthetic or therapeutic environment—is akin to "giving up" on a loved one. The first step to getting unstuck is the caregiver's awareness of the process, of this tug-of-war. Holding on to expectations, resisting change, and working to avoid feelings of loss are normal coping strategies under these frightening circumstances. Only after caregivers become aware of their tug-of-war can they move toward accepting the new reality and developing new coping strategies. This includes recognizing that much of the responsibility for stopping the vicious cycle lies with the caregiver, not the person with dementia.

One caregiver recently said to us with a surprised look on her face, "Oohhh, I get it! You're trying to get *me* to change, not my husband." Because some caregivers may equate responsibility for change with blame, we take care to distinguish the two. A "no fault" rule applies; the current difficulties experienced by both members of the dyad are nobody's fault. Nobody is to blame. That does not mean, however, that the situation cannot be improved. Further, it does not mean that the care recipient is completely let off the hook. Both the caregiver and the person with dementia—particularly when the latter's cognitive impairment is mild—can be "response-able," that is, can be helped to respond in ways that will free the dyad from their trap. To illustrate how this might work, we introduce a new case, that of Mr. Malloy.

CASE 4. MR. MALLOY: HELPING INDIVIDUALS MAINTAIN THEIR LONG-TERM RELATIONSHIPS

Mr. Malloy contacted the regional psychological institute to attend a workshop on anxiety reduction. During the initial screening, 75-year-old Mr. Malloy disclosed that, 1 month previous, he had received a diagnosis of probable Alzheimer's disease. When the intake worker informed him that this diagnosis excluded him from participation in the workshop, Mr. Malloy got angry. He said that he did not know how to keep on living with his spouse, that fear of failure and almost constant criticism and arguments were ruining his life, and that he needed urgent assistance. Mr. Malloy also said he worried about running out of money. The institute's intake worker found that Mr. Malloy represented a moderate to high risk of suicide and referred him to you.

At an in-home assessment, both Mr. Malloy and Mrs. Malloy signed consent forms and provided releases for the exchange of information. Mr. Malloy provided you with copies of his neurological assessments. His MMSE score was 29. He said he was not able to build model cars anymore, his favorite hobby, and had trouble with routine home maintenance. He also described difficulties recalling names and finding his way when leaving his immediate neighborhood.

Mrs. Malloy had a chronic pain condition that prevented her from engaging in many physical activities. Throughout their 10-year marriage, Mr. Malloy had been both provider and caregiver to his wife, a role he clearly valued. Both partners described their initial years together as characterized by respect and affection. Mrs. Malloy, however, felt that in the past year her husband had become "lazy." There had been an increase in arguments that the couple described as "ugly," with mutual accusations on both sides. Mr. Malloy said he worried that because he had always been his wife's caregiver, she might not be able to cope with his new disabilities.

The case of Mr. and Mrs. Malloy differs from previous examples presented in this book. Mr. Malloy represents someone with a recent dementia diagnosis. Although he was clearly experiencing changes in cognitive function, Mr. Malloy had more psychological insight into his situation than persons with more advanced dementia typically do. The case is also unique in that throughout their marriage, Mr. Malloy had been accustomed to being the provider and caregiver, and Mrs. Malloy had expected care. The caregiver–care recipient roles were about to flip-flop, which we might expect could be distressing for both sides. As before, let us think about how functional analysis and use of the DANCE principles might guide your thinking about how best to help this couple.

- D: Discuss concerns respectfully. Because Mr. Malloy's cognitive changes are still mild, it will be not only possible but also important for both members of the couple to be able to discuss their concerns and consider treatment options. How much of the details about his dementia evaluation and diagnosis has Mr. Malloy shared with his wife? Does Mrs. Malloy understand how dementia affects memory, thinking, and motivation? What fears might she have about how she is going to manage if Mr. Malloy is not able to provide the instrumental support she has relied on throughout their marriage?
- A: Ameliorate excess disability. Would the couple benefit from participation in a home care program that could provide physical assistance to Mrs. Malloy or help with home repairs and upkeep? When were Mr. Malloy's most recent medical

checkups? Does he have any concurrent diseases? Is Mrs. Malloy receiving ongoing and appropriate medical follow-up for pain management?

- N: Nurture the dyad. How might we help to restore the mutual affection and respect Mr. and Mrs. Malloy had for each other in the past? Are there activities they could do together that would increase their sense of intimacy and friendship? Would they benefit from communication skill training to help them discuss problems more effectively (rather than using arguing and name-calling)?

- C: Create contextual solutions. Is there a pattern to the couple's arguments? Who initiates them? What do they typically argue about? What does Mrs. Malloy mean when she says that her husband is "lazy"? How do the arguments come to an end? What expectations do they each have for one another, and how have those expectations changed (or not) throughout their marriage?

- E: Enjoy the journey. Does Mr. Malloy have any other hobbies besides building model cars that bring him pleasure? What does his wife do to give her a sense of purpose and satisfaction in spite of her physical limitations? Are there any other family members or friends who are an important part of the couple's lives?

GLOBAL PATTERNS

In our work with Mr. and Mrs. Malloy and other caregiving dyads, we are not interested in analyzing every individual interaction but in detecting global patterns. If we are able to support the caregiver and the person with dementia in identifying multiple instances that fit into a global pattern, we can achieve change on a larger scale. In the case of Mr. and Mrs. Malloy, most of their argumentative encounters revolved around what each was (or was not) doing that made the other person feel less appreciated or valued. Rebuilding the dyadic relationship was a critical piece in helping this couple.

Individuals differ in the circumstances that make them feel loved. Whereas one person may feel loved when a spouse holds open a door, another may feel disrespected and belittled. Although effectively receiving and expressing genuine affection has its ups and downs in all relationships, dementia throws an additional wrench into the system by narrowing what the person with dementia is capable of doing and understanding. Mrs. Malloy felt loved when Mr. Malloy did things for her: driving her, preparing her meals or afternoon tea, or undertaking home maintenance or repair. For his part, Mr. Malloy felt loved when Mrs. Malloy leaned on, needed, and relied on

TABLE 6.1

Overview of the Vicious Cycle in the A • B • Cs for Mr. and Mrs. Malloy

Activators	Mrs. Malloy's behaviors	Consequences
Mr. Malloy ignores his wife's requests for help around the house.	Mrs. Malloy yells.	Mr. Malloy makes vague commitments to do what his wife asked.
Mr. Malloy makes vague commitments to do what his wife asked.	Mrs. Malloy stops yelling.	Mr. Malloy resumes ignoring his wife's requests.
Mr. Malloy resumes ignoring his wife's requests.	Mrs. Malloy yells.	Mr. Malloy makes vague commitment to do what his wife asked (and so on it goes).

him, when she was sweet and appreciative of his task completions. As Mr. Malloy started having difficulties completing complex tasks, his opportunities for showing love decreased. Mrs. Malloy, in turn, did not feel cared for and no longer felt that she could rely on her husband. As a result, she began to engage in behavior that made Mr. Malloy feel unappreciated. Mr. and Mrs. Malloy had entered a coercive vicious cycle: Mrs. Malloy felt that her requests for help around the house remained unheard by Mr. Malloy unless she yelled at him. Mr. Malloy felt that the only way to escape from Mrs. Malloy's constant requests was to give some vague response about future compliance. Both partners felt "trapped." In working with the couple, the behavioral health care specialist was able to present this cycle or "trap" to the couple as a difficulty with the expression and receipt of love rather than an issue about getting household chores done. The chain of A • B • Cs for this ineffective pattern is summarized in Table 6.1.

This particular A • B • C trap is almost ubiquitous in dementia care. Individuals with dementia quickly agree to what a caregiver is asking and thereby escape from the pressures of the caregiver's demands. Then the care recipient finds he or she is unable to start or complete the complex series of steps involved in what he or she has agreed to do. Rather than go to the caregiver and admit this inadequacy, he or she just drops it. Often the caregiver's request gets forgotten altogether.

In working with Mr. and Mrs. Malloy, we brainstormed other opportunities for how each could show how much they cared for each other. One of our hypotheses was that if Mrs. Malloy felt cared for and appreciated, her requests for the completion of complex tasks would decrease. Since we anticipated that Mr. Malloy would have to stop driving in the near future, we focused with Mrs. Malloy on generating a list of simple tasks that Mr. Malloy could complete at home to please her. Their proposed solutions included

(a) hiring a local handyperson whom Mr. Malloy could assist with task completion (Mr. Malloy liked this solution); (b) arranging homemaker services for Mrs. Malloy, so she could request assistance on days she was bedridden; (c) broadening Mrs. Malloy's understanding of dementia-related difficulties in complex task initiation and completion; (d) offering Mrs. Malloy coaching to help her recognize that her husband's attempts to complete simple tasks are a reflection of his love for her; (e) supporting Mr. Malloy by validating his concerns about the diagnosis and the concurrent loss of his caregiver and provider role; and (f) working with both spouses to generate acceptance of feelings of frustration, sadness, anger, guilt, and other emotions evoked by the degenerative and incurable disease.

We found that Mr. Malloy's feelings of hopelessness and worthlessness were a direct function of his spouse's reactions to his inability to initiate or carry out his usual chores, rather than a function of clinical depression. Once Mrs. Malloy understood that Mr. Malloy deeply cared for her but was increasingly limited in how he could demonstrate this affection, she began to acknowledge his simple task attempts and completions, and their arguments decreased and marital satisfaction increased. Continuing homework to identify and engage in simple activities that both spouses enjoyed also enriched their relationship.

PRESERVING IMPORTANT ROLE IDENTITIES

Although many functional roles change as dementia progresses, it is important to preserve care recipients' key role identities as long as possible, both as a way of demonstrating respect for the individual with dementia and to help caregivers maintain a balanced perspective on their relationship with the care recipient. Our intervention with Mr. and Mrs. Malloy targeted alternative ways to help both spousal partners feel loved and appreciated. They valued that they were contributing to the relationship as equals. In child–parent relationships we often search for ways that adult children can provide care without starting to treat the parent like a child. One family, for example, was concerned about how Dad would be able to attend a holiday gathering if he could not remember anybody's names or follow conversations. The adult children decided they would create a special seat for Dad, in the middle of the gathering, where he would give out all of the Christmas presents, labeled with each person's name. The father was thus able to graciously bestow gifts upon all attendees, was never in the awkward position of having to remember a name or a face, and earned a lot of smiles, thank yous, hugs, kisses, and general appreciation. How different would things have turned out if he had attended the gathering expected to know and interact with a plethora of people he could not place into context? Thanks to the family's advanced strategizing, the father's role as the patriarch of the family was preserved.

By using the A • B • Cs to consider a person's important life roles within their larger psychosocial context, we can actively help persons with dementia maintain their relationships and personal identity at the same time we provide needed assistive care. Here are some more examples:

- Mrs. Smith, whom you came to know in Chapter 3, used to be a nurse. During doctors' visits, she gladly collaborated with requests if she was asked to assist: "Could you help me take your blood pressure, please?"

- Mr. Norfolk received a Presidential Early Career Award for Scientists and Engineers. Although he did not remember the specifics of his work, he liked recalling the joyous excitement of traveling to the White House and attending the award ceremony. His son found that saying, "A person is coming to interview you about the White House ceremony" facilitated Mr. Norfolk's acceptance of agency-based respite care workers.

- Mr. Glasure used to be a project manager for an international building contractor. Staff members of the specialized dementia care unit where he resided provided him with a walkie-talkie in the morning. He went to work, attended staff meetings, and related to staff members as their project manager. With Mr. Glasure's "employment," elopement attempts decreased.

- Angie found that her mom's mood considerably improved in the morning after Angie put her in charge of the morning coffee. Angie prepared mugs with water and instant coffee in advance, so her mom only had to push a big red dot on the microwave for a 1-minute reheat and then serve the coffee to Angie.

- Zoe's mother, Soula, used to instruct her daughter in crafts. Soula was quite a perfectionist and virtually stopped engaging in any activity when her motor skills started failing her. Then Zoe discovered new coloring booklets with a cloth-like texture, designed for adults. Small velvet boundaries kept Soula's coloring markers within the lines, so each coloring could be perfect. Soula now colors several hours per day and regularly gives Zoe advice on how to color.

- Jonathan's father, Edgar, lives with Jonathan and his wife. Although Edgar lost most of his savings in the stock market crash and relies on Social Security and his son's support, he tells visitors that the home is his and that he has graciously allowed Jonathan and his family to move in with him. Jonathan and his wife, Margaret, do not dispute Edgar's narrative; instead, they add statements of how lucky they are to have a dad such as Edgar.

As increasing numbers of baby boomers with unconventional lifestyles and preferences become the care recipients, there will be a growing need to find nontraditional and creative ways to preserve role identities and relationships. For example, broad-based dementia education programs may spur new models of communal or multigenerational living that allow individuals with dementia to be part of everyday life (i.e., do communally what they are still able to do) without becoming stigmatized as "old," "senile," or "crotchety." Rather than isolating individuals with cognitive impairment and providing custodial care, such communal living models could resemble an old-fashioned neighborhood of people committed to each others' care, not unlike existing nonprofit Quaker retirement villages but multigenerational in nature. Alternatively, education and social acceptance could foster opportunities for volunteerism in which even persons with moderate cognitive impairment could feel like they have an active role and are contributing to the greater good around them. In lieu of these perhaps utopian living arrangements, the better you know your client, the more efficient you will be in coaching caregivers to interact in a way that maintains what the person with dementia used to value and that helps his or her current sense of self be protected and preserved.

PICKING PRIORITIES: BEING "RIGHT" OR
HAVING A GOOD RELATIONSHIP

The examples presented earlier illustrate that nurturing the dyad means sometimes suspending factual accuracy and listening to the heart of the relationship rather than to the voice of reason. Many caregivers just want the care recipient to "snap out of it," to "tell the truth," or "stop acting crazy." Because most of our clients are people of honesty, integrity, and reason, caregivers' dislike of either the care recipients' or their own behaviors that seem dishonest, inconsistent, or downright silly is understandable. Nevertheless, overt efforts to change what a person with dementia thinks, feels, or does seldom, or never, work. Often, they only make matters worse. For this reason, we ask caregivers to make the sometimes unimaginable leap to truly be with the person with dementia and with whatever he or she brings to the table. People with dementia are struggling to maintain their relationship networks and a sense of belonging. Many caregivers think the way to help people with dementia do that is to fight their disease symptoms and to orient them to reality, no matter what. In contrast, we focus on helping caregivers to "accept the things they cannot change," hypothesizing what might pragmatically "work" in each unique situation, and monitoring whether new strategies bring the caregiver and care recipient closer.

For example, many persons with dementia have a fluid conception of time. Our clients often cannot fathom themselves being older than 40 or appreciate that it is the 21st century. Given the age and time distortion, there can be considerable confusion as to the identity of family members: Paid caregivers may be wives, daughters may be sisters, husbands may be fathers, sons may be college friends. If gentle attempts at correction fail, then we recommend that all efforts to convince, persuade, correct, plead, or right a wrong be abandoned. Continued change efforts may set up a history of interpersonal conflict that leaves the person with dementia fearful, apprehensive, or mistrustful of the caregiver. Humorously, sometimes care recipients' misidentifications reveal aspects of ourselves that we might not want to see, as in the case of a woman with dementia who calls her husband by the name of her stern and corrective father. One caregiver told us that after she uncharacteristically lost her temper with her husband, he commented, "I want the nice lady who visits me to come back tomorrow." Our clients' observations thus often tell us what needs to be done to preserve the dyadic relationship, and how important this relationship is to them.

THIRD-PARTY ASSISTANCE

Some of the caregivers with whom we work have cared for their spouses or parents since the early 1990s, a stretch of almost 2 decades. They have learned to think and plan for two, have given up most of their leisure activities, restricted contact with their friends, and focused their whole being on keeping the person with dementia engaged. A few caregivers care for two people: mother and husband, brother and wife. Unfortunately, such singular dedication can take its toll on the caregiver's health; sleep deprivation, constant worry about the loved one's safety and comfort, and lack of self-care (e.g., exercise, medical checkups) are all common consequences.

Ironically, this level of devotion is not usually best for the care recipient either. What would happen to the person with dementia if the caregiver fell ill? How would he or she cope with a transition to other caregivers who might not be familiar with established routines? Some self-protective behaviors such as striking out serve an anxiety-reducing function and can be avoided by gently exposing the care recipient to multiple individuals (such as in an adult day program) rather than a single round-the-clock caregiver. It is notable that many people with dementia thrive once they break out of an isolating dyadic relationship; they enjoy activities in adult day programs, have fun visiting with family, and even do well on respite stays in nearby residential care settings.

Coaching caregivers to accept third-party assistance can be challenging, however. Caregivers are often correct when they say that their quality of care can never be replicated by a paid professional. Third-party assistance also creates its own additional stressors and burdens that in some situations become the "straw that breaks the camel's back." Having another person with different habits and routines sharing your household can be difficult. Aides may be competent but a poor cultural or personality match for the care recipient or family caregiver. Disasters do occasionally occur when the third party's background and references are not carefully checked. Professional caregiving can also be expensive. Ironically, many caregivers receive an allocation of respite funds from community agencies yet do not use the moneys because they consider themselves not quite "there" or not "desperate enough," and they fear their loved one's resistance to in-home help. In our practice we spend much time educating caregivers about the proper use and benefits of assistance. For example, we preselect and suggest respite options, educate in-home health professionals hired by the family, accompany family caregivers to intake appointments at residential respite care facilities, validate and address concerns, monitor the care recipient's respite experience, and solve problems with the caregiver if care was perceived as inadequate. Concurrently, we assist caregivers in rebuilding a life with other extended family and friends.

EXPANDING THE COMMUNITY OF FAMILY CARE

Reestablishing a life that includes others and not just the person with dementia is problematic for some caregivers. Many do not feel understood by family or friends who fail to grasp the complexities of genuinely caring for somebody with progressive, degenerative dementia. Well-meaning attempts at helping ("Why don't you just . . . ?") may feel dismissive and invalidate the complex nature of dementia care. Depending on the assessment of the caregiver's relationships with family and friends, an intervention may target the building of interpersonal skills to repair relationships with siblings, parents, or friends who have drifted out of the supportive network of care. We have conducted family education and support sessions to offer opportunities for family inclusion. Often, these family sessions reveal that other family members and friends feel they were "shut out" or criticized as "not good enough" to be of assistance when they failed to anticipate some of the care recipient's needs or made an inadvertent comment that turned the caregiver away from relying on them as a resource. "You just don't understand," is an isolating and recurrent thought for many caregivers. For some caregivers, it is also difficult to let go and discover that the care recipient can do well under someone else's care; like Mr. Malloy, they feel loved when they are needed. Such caregivers can feel devastated when the care recipient does not recognize them after a weeklong absence. A successful intervention for extended social support has to address these feelings of loss.

COMPLEX FAMILY SITUATIONS

It is not unusual to meet caregiver dyads who were having serious relationship problems prior to one of the partners receiving a formal dementia diagnosis. Care recipients with forms of dementia (e.g., frontotemporal) that impact judgment and impulse control are particularly likely to engage in activities that fracture relationships. They may overspend their budget, engage in unusual risk-taking, have sex with people other than their usual partner, or leave their spouses altogether. Once the dementia diagnosis is made, some spouses and adult children feel a moral obligation to care for the care recipient. This can be either a good or a bad decision. In some cases, the dementia diagnosis provides an explanation for many baffling and infuriating care recipient behaviors, and the dyadic relationship may actually improve. As the caregiver learns how to communicate more effectively, interactions become easier and regain some of their reinforcing aspects, such as expressions of affection, trust, and laughter. Personality changes can make care recipients more compliant and agreeable than before dementia onset. Relationships that had struggled under the burden of old hurts and grievances can begin to blossom when the person with dementia no longer remembers what she was angry about or no longer recognizes the person who had wronged her long ago.

Unfortunately, mutual expectations and the tug-of-war described earlier usually make the interactions between caregiver and care recipient more difficult rather than easier. Providing care for a person one may not trust, like, or respect for historical reasons requires a level of detachment that is beyond most people's skills. Some studies suggest that nearly a third of family members caring for persons with dementia report acting abusively toward them (Selwood, Cooper, Owens, Blanchard, & Livingston, 2009). Spouses or adult children with a long history of conflict with the care recipient may need to make the difficult decision to step away from being a primary caregiver. Spouses in their 40s and 50s, asked to provide full-time care for a partner while still raising small children or pursuing a career may have neither the time nor energy available to provide good dementia care. If differences are irreconcilable, health care professionals can facilitate the transition to another more appropriate primary caregiver, perhaps another family member, public guardian, or long-term residential care setting. Given the detrimental effects of ongoing and irreconcilable interpersonal conflict, this transition is also in the best interest of the person with dementia. Once new or professional caregivers oversee and provide care, it becomes possible to turn time-limited visitations between the former caregiver and the care recipient into pleasant and relationship-building occasions.

SEXUAL BEHAVIOR

Sexual behavior is a powerful source of mutual pleasure; regardless of age, it usually only decreases in frequency because of lack of opportunity (e.g., death of a spouse) or physical disability and chronic ailment (Lindau et al., 2007). Some couples experience mutual sexual fulfillment for years in the presence of cognitive decline, whereas others do not. For example, Mr. and Mrs. Malloy's sexual relationship had ceased some years ago because of Mrs. Malloy's chronic pain condition. Advancing dementia also eventually undermines the desire and ability to engage in mutually satisfying sexual intercourse. Some cognitively impaired individuals find sexual contact to be anxiety provoking and do not understand what their caregivers are asking them to do. Caregivers sometimes feel awkward or uncomfortable engaging in sexual activity when their spouse is too cognitively impaired to remember the intimate encounter later. Other caregivers would like to continue sexual relations but cease them because of their loved one's failing health. These caregivers may benefit from learning to separate physical intimacy and sexual experiences and from learning how to generate intimacy in the absence of sex. Holding hands, snuggling, cuddling, spending time in bed together, and other forms of simple sexual play are all nonverbal means that preserve an important aspect of the couple's past relationship and can be gratifying to caregiving dyads. When providing services to couples, it is important to assess their current sexual functioning and expectations because they might affect the degree of interpersonal distress and conflict experienced.

Accusations of Infidelity

Accusations of infidelity are common as people with dementia try to make sense of changes in the quality of their marital relationships. In our practice, we have observed individuals with dementia who accuse their spouses of infidelity when sexual relations decline. Because the care recipient lacks insight into the underlying physical and cognitive causes, the decline

TABLE 6.2

Sample Overview of the A • B • Cs for Accusations of Infidelity

Activators	Behaviors	Consequences
Cessation of sexual intercourse Absence of physical affection Spouse often frowning, correcting, chiding Spouse frequently talking to other people Spouse absent for unexplained periods of time	Accusing spouse of having an extramarital affair	Spouse reassures with physical affection. Spouse reassures by saying, "I love you." Spouse stops talking to others.
Broader psychosocial context: History of infidelity in family	*Gather a behavioral history:* Gradual worsening in marital relationship accompanies increasing cognitive decline.	*Conduct a general reinforcer assessment:* Feeling loved and cherished by caregiver

seems "out of the blue" and leads him or her to the conclusion that the spouse must be having an affair. Care recipients who are left alone and forget that the caregiver said she was going shopping or having lunch with a friend also sometimes fill in the unexplained absence with suspicions that the caregiver is meeting a lover. Assessment of marital history is imperative because there may have been infidelity in the care recipient's life—sometimes indirectly, as when a person's mother may have left the father for another man. Historical factors combined with an absence of physical affection and verbally or non-verbally expressed criticism (e.g., frowning, correcting, chiding) all can set the occasion for accusations of infidelity.

Accusations of infidelity, like all verbal behavior, can be difficult to change because they can serve multiple important functions. For example, accusations can be a way of making sense out of the otherwise unexplainable changes in the caregiver's behavior (*activators* in Table 6.2). The accusations may also be indirect requests for attention, romantic interludes, or physical contact that the caregiver inadvertently reinforces by her attempts to reassure the cognitively impaired spouse (*consequences* in Table 6.2). In one possible intervention, you could work with the spouse to offer affection and reassurance multiple times during the day noncontingently (i.e., only at times when the accusatory behavior does not occur). This example intervention does not question the need for intimacy and affection, yet makes the behavior that has been the gateway to need fulfillment unnecessary.

Institutionalization, Sex, and Intimacy

Sexual needs and desires can lead to a set of entirely different problems when the individual with dementia moves to a dementia care unit.[2] There, increased confusion and behavioral disinhibition may lead to physical encounters, including disrobing in public, touching self or others, sexual talk or masturbation, or sexual intercourse with other residents. Although sexual behaviors are rare, when they occur they tend to be upsetting to staff members and family. As with all behaviors of persons with dementia, a functional analysis using the A • B • Cs should be conducted. What was the behavior of concern? Was it verbal (e.g., "You look pretty today," "I bet you would like a boyfriend") or nonverbal (e.g., touching, grabbing)? Is this a new behavior or an ongoing or worsening pattern? What are possible activators? Has the staff member misinterpreted an erection during genital care as a sexual advance? Has there been a change in medications? Does the resident have a urinary tract infection? Could the behavior be a reflection of unmet needs for intimacy? Persons with dementia who have continued to be sexually active at home and now are moved into a residence away from their spouse might experience the sudden change in physical closeness acutely. Even if the person with dementia has not been sexually active for some time, individuals who have never slept alone since childhood may attempt to climb into bed with other residents. Individuals seeking intimacy and connection are by far more common than those seeking sexual relationships. When intimate behaviors between residents occur, such as holding hands, embracing, or sitting closely, the effect on the spousal caregiver may not be much different in kind from having to cope with an extramarital affair of a sexual nature. Adult children who recall their parents' relationship as dedicated and singular can also struggle with the presence of another woman or man in their parent's life. As health care providers, we can help caregivers understand that these behaviors are not a rejection of the person's life partner; rather, as verbal skills fail, connection to others can sometimes only be maintained through such nonverbal, physical means. For example, when Supreme Court Justice Sandra Day O'Connor learned that her husband of over 50 years, who had Alzheimer's disease, had developed an emotional attachment to another resident in his nursing care facility, she accepted this as a part of the disease. Justice O'Connor's compas-

---

[2]Sexual disinhibition or hypersexuality can also occur in persons with cognitive impairment who are still living in the community. For a more thorough discussion of particular symptoms as well as pharmacological and nonpharmacological approaches to its management, see Wallace and Safer (2009). From the A • B • C perspective, antecedents and consequences that usually govern proper conduct lose their effectiveness in persons with dementia, resulting in sexual behavior that occurs "at the wrong place and time." Commonly used anxiolytic drugs, such as benzodiazepines, may cause or exacerbate the problem (McKim, 2003; Poling & Byrne, 2000).

sionate response was exemplary of the acceptance and openness to the sometimes painful change that should be nurtured among our clients and their families.

Many facilities and staff, however, will not tolerate any physical contact between residents. Ageism is prevalent around issues of sexuality, and many workable solutions in dementia care fall outside of the current social norms (e.g., permitting sexual relations or intimacy between residents who are married to other people). Residents who seek out physical companionship with other residents are often labeled as sexually aggressive perpetrators, discharged from the facility, or treated with drugs commonly used for sexual offenders (e.g., hormone treatment). Family members can find that care recipients who have been transferred out of residential care for this reason may be blackballed from entry anywhere else. Our work as health care providers includes facilitating open communication around sexual issues with the caregiver and the facility. Many factors need to be considered. Are the activities consensual, and are both parties capable of giving informed consent? Has the spouse/family/guardian of the involved residents been informed and given consent? Is there monitoring for sexual health and sexually transmitted diseases? Is privacy available to residents and actually provided in the care facility? Are residents permitted to continue sexual relations with visiting spouses? How should facility policies deal with staff caregivers whose personal or cultural value systems strongly oppose sexual contact of any type between residents? What assessment and notification procedures are in place to ensure that everyone's safety and rights are protected?

Functional analysis and use of the A • B • Cs can be extremely useful in helping facilities think through their general policies on sexuality as well as solve problems about individual resident behaviors (see Table 6.3). As health care professionals, we are poised to assist in this dialogue. We strongly recommend obtaining releases for the exchange of information and including professional caregivers as well as family, physicians, and administration in the educational and problem-solving processes.

PUTTING THE CONTEXTUAL MODEL TO WORK

Nurturing the dyad is a complex process that requires us to abandon preconceived notions about individuals with dementia, aging, and relationships. It asks us to think creatively, notice our judgments and evaluations (e.g., if a spouse or daughter decides not to function as a primary caregiver), and consistently strive to establish a community of genuine care. In this chapter, we have seen that the contextual model of care can be as useful for supporting this community of care as it is for solving specific behavioral problems. In

TABLE 6.3

Example of How A • B • Cs Can Be Used to Think about
Sexuality Policies in Long-Term Care

Activators	Behaviors	Consequences
Boredom and inactivity	Sexual behaviors:	Calm, matter of fact
Uncomfortable clothing	• Disrobing in public	response
Room temperature	• Touching self or others	Use of simple instructions
Loneliness, depression,	• Sex talk	Clear limit-setting
or anxiety	• Crawling into bed with	Staff avoid flirtatious/joking
Changes in medications	other residents	behavior
Urinary or bowel infection	• Use of pornography	Notification of family, staff
or incontinence	• Masturbation	administration, physician
Misinterpretation of staff	• Attempts at intercourse	Careful record keeping:
personal care activities		• Date, location, witnesses,
Expressive aphasia,		previous patterns
agnosia		• Rationale for medication
Vision impairment		management and
		restrictive clothing
		Staff educational focus
		groups
		Establishment of private
		spaces for capable
		residents
Broader psychosocial *context:*		*Conduct a general reinforcer* *assessment:*
• Recent move from home with spouse.		• Use of touch to feel loved and cherished.
• Sexual orientation.		
• Lifelong attitudes toward nudity and personal hygiene.		
• History of sexual abuse or assault.		

Chapter 7, we examine the evidence-based support for the contextual model and see how it compares with other empirical treatments that have been developed for working with cognitively impaired persons and their caregivers. By doing so, we hope to enrich your ability to create contextual solutions that are efficacious in whatever health care role or dementia care setting you may find yourselves.

7

CREATE CONTEXTUAL SOLUTIONS: MANAGING COMMON AFFECTIVE AND BEHAVIORAL CHANGES

Many of the strategies outlined so far—discussing concerns respectfully, ameliorating excess disability, and nurturing the dyad—can be preventive in nature. Honoring our clients' preferences, managing conditions that worsen cognitive symptoms, and helping restore and preserve valued relationships reduce much of the suffering associated with a dementia diagnosis. As the aging population becomes more "psychologically minded" and early diagnoses more common, there are increasing numbers of persons with dementia, like Mr. Malloy, who initiate their own supportive services and treatments. Much of the health care professional's work with such clients is to help them to understand their diagnosis, evaluate their treatment options, and make decisions about the future that are consistent with their values and preferences. Although advance planning for a life with progressive, degenerative dementia can be difficult and heart-wrenching in the short term, in the long run such planning is easier than ignoring the problem and being caught off guard by the inevitable decline. We cannot overstate the importance of foresight.

The majority of our clients, however, are not self-referred. Rather, they are those in later stages of dementia, such as Mrs. Flynn, Mrs. Smith, and Mrs. Puttani, who are brought to our attention by agencies or caregivers bewildered by the care recipient's pronounced mood and behavioral changes.

In these cases, our task is to help caregivers develop creative, flexible, and individualized problem-solving strategies that will get the situation "unstuck." A contextual approach is ideally suited to the task. However, because the contextual model addresses patterns and functions of behavior rather than offering a specific solution to particular symptoms, implementation requires looking at multiple examples and repeated observations. This is a process that can take a while to learn and some considerable practice, whereas patients with dementia and caregivers often need help addressing behavioral problems right away. In this chapter, we describe some alternative approaches to dementia care that can give you ideas on how to "jump-start" the problem-solving process using concepts that will seem familiar and reasonable to most clients. We also consider in what ways these alternative approaches are compatible with the contextual model described throughout this book, and how they might enrich your contextual problem-solving skills.

IMPLEMENT NONPHARMACOLOGICAL SOLUTIONS: THE FIRST-LINE RECOMMENDATION

It is important to begin by remembering that nondrug interventions are not a last resort or fallback alternative for dealing with thorny dementia-related behavioral challenges. Several international and national professional associations and government policies have recommended nonpharmacological interventions as the first-line treatment for the affective and behavioral changes associated with dementia (American Geriatrics Society and American Association for Geriatric Psychiatry, 2003a, 2003b; Doody et al., 2001; Lyketsos et al., 2006; Small et al., 1997). In U.S. nursing homes, the Nursing Home Reform Act, passed as part of the Omnibus Budget Reconciliation Act (1987), mandates the documented trial of a nonpharmacological intervention before considering drug treatments for neuropsychiatric symptoms in nursing home residents.[1] In practice, however, medications are widely viewed as the primary treatment for mood and behavioral changes in persons with dementia, and many persons referred to you will be treated using one or more antidepressant, anxiolytic, antipsychotic, and/or sleeping medications before a nonpharmacological intervention is tried.

There is currently no absolute standard of care for the pharmacological management of neuropsychiatric symptoms of dementia. Medication treatment effects are modest, side effect risks are significant, and because of their

---

[1]The Omnibus Budget Reconciliation Act (1987) in Federal Regulations 42 C.F.R. 483.25 describes the requirements for enhancing quality of care in long term care facilities (available from the Government Printing Office at http://www.gpo.gov/).

adverse risk potential, some medications (e.g., long-acting benzodiazepines, antipsychotics) should be avoided altogether except for short-term or occasional use.[2] Use of drugs to stop one behavior that is a "problem" can also inadvertently affect other behaviors that you would like to see maintained. For example, a person who is engaging in repetitive verbalizations may stop repeating the same phrase (e.g., "Help me!") over and over but may also lose the ability to ask for anything else he or she wants or may become incontinent and prone to falls. Preservation of remaining abilities is precious to persons living with a progressive neurodegenerative disease. Thus, although nonpharmacological interventions are not "magic bullets" that will immediately eliminate every problem that comes your way, they should always be considered and tried first.

OVERVIEW OF NONPHARMACOLOGICAL INTERVENTIONS FOR BEHAVIORAL AND AFFECTIVE CHANGES

When you search the literature for approaches to reducing behavioral and affective changes in dementia, you will find three main categories of evidence-based interventions. Interventions that overlap most closely with the contextual model followed in this book include those also known as *social learning, behavior management, operant,* or *behavioral* treatments. Common to all of these is their use of an ABC approach and their use of key behavioral principles such as reinforcement. These interventions are not solely intended for application with persons with dementia and their caregivers; A • B • C analyses can be and are used to study and treat a wide variety of behaviors and clinical populations across the age span.[3]

In addition to the contextual model, two other theoretically based approaches to dementia care have been systematically evaluated: (a) the *need-driven dementia-compromised behavior* approach (NDB; Algase et al., 1996) and (b) the *environmental vulnerability* or *progressively lowered stress threshold* model (PLST; Cohen-Mansfield, 2000; Hall, 1994; Hall & Buckwalter, 1987; Smith, Gerdner, Hall, & Buckwalter, 2004; Smith, Hall, Gerdner, & Buckwalter,

---

[2]For discussion of the effects of drugs on geriatric populations and, in particular, concerns about the use of psychotropic medications to manage neuropsychiatric changes in dementia, see Salzman (2005); Sink, Holden, and Yaffe (2005); and "Treatment of Agitation" (1998). Also, see Chapter 5, footnotes 2 and 3.
[3]Behavior analytic tools have long been the mainstay of treating autism spectrum disorders or other developmental disabilities in children and adults. More pertinent to adult and geriatric populations, many cognitive rehabilitative techniques apply the contextual model in the form of complex antecedent and consequent interventions. For example, for patients who are post-head injury or stroke, behavioral and affective changes can often be reduced or avoided altogether by using an A • B • C approach to create individualized prosthetic and supportive environments to compensate for cognitive deficits. For further information, see Sohlberg and Mateer (2001) and Wesolowski and Zencius (1994).

2006). The NDB and PLST explanatory frameworks originally emerged to train professional caregivers working with severely cognitively impaired individuals in long-term care settings. The basic assumptions of the NDB and PLST approaches, compared with the contextual model, can be summarized as follows:

- Contextual model: As activators and consequences are altered, all individuals' emotions, thoughts, and actions change over time in ways predicted and influenced by A • B • C principles.
- NDB: All people, regardless of dementia severity, have basic needs. A person's increasing inability to communicate these needs leads to affective and behavioral changes.
- PLST: Neurodegenerative decline sensitizes individuals to the effects of stress. The accumulation of psychosocial stressors increases the likelihood of affective and behavioral reactions.

All three intervention approaches share the view that mood and behavior changes are "normal" consequences of cognitive impairment rather than aberrant neuropsychiatric "symptoms." Indeed, the three explanatory frameworks are complementary on many levels, as can be seen in Exhibit 7.1. Given their many similarities, all three explanatory frameworks can be useful for

EXHIBIT 7.1
Similarities Among NDB, PLST, and Contextual Model Approaches to Managing Mood and Behavioral Changes in Persons With Dementia

- All shift the focus from pejorative labeling of neuropsychiatric symptoms as "problems" to seeing affective and behavioral changes as compensatory or communicative phenomena that can be understood and responded to in a manner that improves a client's quality of life.
- All are based on the larger notion of person–environment fit.
- All emphasize the importance of considering both an individual's past as well as current circumstances in understanding the development and maintenance of affective and behavioral changes.
- All emphasize the importance of the dyadic interaction between client and caregiver.
- All emphasize the importance of decreased verbal communication as an underlying cause of mood and behavioral changes.
- All have theory-based explanations for why these mood and behavioral changes escalate or de-escalate over time.
- All emphasize that effective treatment requires responding to the underlying need or broader context, not just eliminating the "symptom" of concern.
- All recommend use of behavioral logs to identify psychosocial, affective, or behavioral patterns.

Note. The conceptual comparison among the NDB, and PLST, and learning and behavioral approaches to dementia care was first laid out by Cohen-Mansfield (2000) and has since been used to provide structure to other reviews of evidence-based treatments for neuropsychiatric symptoms in persons with dementia (Ayalon, Gum, Felician, & Arean, 2006; Logsdon, McCurry, & Teri, 2007). NDB = need-driven dementia-compromised behavior; PLST = progressively lowered stress threshold.

health care professionals who wish to help caregivers understand the context in which mood or behavioral changes develop. Caregiver skills training takes time and effort, and caregiver acceptance of your rationale and treatment approach is essential. Incorporating NDB and PLST concepts into your problem-solving approach can increase caregiver buy-in because these models offer everyday explanations of behavior to which we all can relate (e.g., not getting what one wants or needs and being stressed). PLST's emphasis on addressing safety concerns and environmental stressors, and the NDB focus on client needs (e.g., hunger, relief from pain), can also help caregivers brainstorm activators and consequences that are important within the A • B • C framework. However, implementing a full A • B • C functional analysis will often still be important sooner or later, when recalcitrant or intractable problems are encountered that persist even after excess disability and overwhelming psychosocial situations have been addressed. For this reason, many psychoeducational interventions for dementia caregivers are multicomponent treatments that guide them to rule out client needs, overwhelming demands, and excess disability while teaching behavioral management within an A • B • C framework.[4]

APPLYING THE CONTEXTUAL MODEL TO SPECIFIC BEHAVIOR CHALLENGES

For the remainder of this chapter, we use clinical examples to illustrate how the contextual model can be used to treat four common categories of mood and behavior changes in dementia: (a) depression and anxiety, (b) agitation and aggression, (c) wandering and circadian rhythm disturbances, and (d) erroneous beliefs and accusatory behaviors. For each problem category, we present a clinical example and describe how NDB or PLST concepts might assist caregivers as they consider possible activators and consequences for behavior and solve treatment strategy problems.

Depression and Anxiety in Dementia: Mr. Smith

Mr. Smith is a 69-year-old man, diagnosed 2 years ago with Alzheimer's disease. His caregiver is his 65-year-old wife. He retired from his job as

---

[4]Many caregiver training programs, such as the Resources for Enhancing Alzheimer's Caregiver Health studies, are multicomponent programs that include a combination of education about strategies for managing neuropsychiatric changes in persons with dementia, and tools to help caregivers improve their own mood, reduce stress, and increase knowledge of and access to community resources (Cooke, McNally, Mulligan, Harrison, & Newman, 2001). Most are explicitly based on cognitive–behavioral treatments, but their conceptualization of care recipient behaviors often are more eclectic and overlap with other theories such as the PLST and need-based models. Reviews of the caregiver treatment literature can be found in Brodaty, Green, and Koschera (2003); Schulz et al. (2002); and Zarit and Femia (2008).

an electrician at age 65 and reportedly had few interests outside of work. When you first see him, you learn that over the past 6 months Mr. Smith has become increasingly withdrawn, avoiding social activities such as church functions and his grandchildren's sports events. Mr. Smith complains of feeling restless, and his wife confirms that he paces about the house, following her around as she tries to do her chores and hobbies. She also says that he has episodes of tearfulness that he finds embarrassing, and he tells her, "I'm no good to anyone anymore." Mrs. Smith herself reports frequent crying spells, disrupted sleep, weight gain, and feelings of hopelessness, largely related to the couple's increasing isolation and to her concern about her husband, who has been resistant to her attempts to get him out of the house and doing things again.

This is a case in which not only is the care recipient with dementia struggling with depression but the caregiver is also presenting with clear depressive symptoms. This is common when working with community-dwelling dyads. Thus, the best intervention for couples such as this would be one that could target depression in both the caregiver and care recipient. A depression treatment program that has been developed as part of the Seattle Protocols meets this criterion.

The *Seattle Protocols* are a group of manualized, evidence-based interventions that provide caregiver education about dementia and realistic expectations, training in effective communication and the A • B • C model of behavior change, assistance identifying and engaging caregivers and care recipients in higher levels of meaningful and pleasurable activities, and information about community resources such as caregiver respite and adult day programs (Teri, Logsdon, & McCurry, 2005). Each protocol also focuses on a specific behavioral challenge and care environment; for example, treatment of depression in community-based settings.[5]

In the Seattle Protocols depression treatment program, caregivers are taught that depression is caused by a decrease in meaningful life activities and an increase in unpleasant person–environment interactions. As the number of pleasant and meaningful activities and interactions declines, a person becomes more withdrawn and apathetic, leading to further withdrawal from participation in pleasant and meaningful activities, and so on goes the depressive spiral. Conversely, increases in meaningful activity (i.e., positive rein-

---

[5]For further explication of the theory underlying treatment of depression in persons with dementia, and for details about the Seattle Protocols depression treatment, see Teri (1994); Teri and Logsdon (1991); and Teri, Logsdon, Uomoto, and McCurry (1997). Treatment descriptions and outcome data based on the Seattle Protocols targeting a variety of other clinical populations, residential care settings, and neuropsychiatric symptoms are available in Logsdon et al. (2010); McCurry, Gibbons, Logsdon, Vitiello, and Teri (2005); McCurry, LaFazia, Pike, Logsdon, and Teri (2009); P.H. Mitchell et al. (2009); Teri et al. (2003); Teri, Huda, Gibbons, Young, and van Leynseele (2005); Teri, Logsdon, and McCurry (2005, 2008); Teri, McCurry, Logsdon, and Gibbons (2005); and Teri et al. (2000).

forcement) lead to an increase in positive affect and behavior, even when the person has dementia.[6] Table 7.1 illustrates how this cycle is played out in the case of Mr. Smith. We can see in Table 7.1 that although the NDB and PSLT models were not developed for use with individuals with mild dementia or community-dwelling individuals, the concepts of client needs and environmental stressors fit nicely into the larger psychosocial context in Mr. Smith's A • B • C analysis. They can also help with problem-solving strategies to improve the situation. For example, pleasant event planning with this couple might include activities specifically aimed at Mr. Smith's needs, such as identifying ways that he could still be helpful around the house.

It is important to note that the A • B • Cs could also be used to guide and help Mrs. Smith. Although she has been well intentioned, her responses to her husband's depressive behaviors have functioned to increase his feelings of worthlessness and to further isolate the couple from family and friends. One strength of the contextual model of dementia care is that it focuses on not just activators for behavior but also on the consequent end of the A • B • C framework. Many caregivers, like Mrs. Smith, do not realize that care recipients are often unable to initiate and follow through with pleasant, meaningful activities on their own. This couple would be helped to identify and engage in pleasant events that they could do together and that would be appropriate given Mr. Smith's level of cognitive decline. Other caregivers are not able to identify what would bring the care recipient pleasure and are surprised by the fun they can both have in new situations. (The process of identifying and implementing pleasant events is described in greater detail in Chapter 8.) Treatment could also help Mrs. Smith alter her punishing verbal responses to her husband, find structured dementia-appropriate programs that could engage him in enjoyable activities, and identify family and friends who could regularly spend time with Mr. Smith so his wife could have some separate quality time on her own. Obstacles to implementing these planned changes would then be anticipated and addressed by using the A • B • Cs.

Agitation and Aggression in Dementia: Mrs. Jones

Mrs. Jones is 79 years old and is cared for by her 80-year-old husband. Before they retired, Mrs. Jones worked as a housekeeper. Her husband was a security guard and still works part time as a school crossing guard. Mr. and Mrs. Jones have both been your clients for 10 years. She has hypertension but is otherwise physically healthy; he has diabetes and

---

[6]Meaningful activity as an antidote to depression was initially proposed by Ferster (1973) and later elaborated by Lewinsohn and colleagues in their Coping with Depression course (Lewinsohn, Antonuccio, Steinmetz, & Teri, 1984; Lewinsohn & Graf, 1973). A contemporary guide for practitioners, particularly relevant to the work with caregivers, is Martell, Addis, and Jacobson (2001).

TABLE 7.1
Using the A • B • Cs to Understand Mr. Smith's Depression and Anxiety

Activators	Behaviors	Consequences
Boredom and inactivity Embarrassment about his emotions Loss of connection with friends and family Progressive loss of skills	Depressive behaviors: • Refusing to participate in previously pleasurable events • Crying • Saying, "I'm worthless" or "I'm of no use" Anxiety behaviors: • Complaining of restlessness • Pacing • Following the caregiver	Isolation and avoidance of psychosocial demands Engaging intensively with Mrs. Smith Mrs. Smith urging him to get out and do more Mrs. Smith suggesting past activities ("Why don't you . . . ?") Mrs. Smith spending more time alone with her husband Mrs. Smith feeling helpless, impatient, and overwhelmed
Broader psychosocial context: Retirement a few years ago Medical context: Neurodegenerative disease Basic "needs": Respect from other people Feeling useful Wanting to be a good husband Stressors: Fatigue and inactivity Loss of work routine and companionship Mrs. Smith urging her husband to get out and do more	*Gather a behavioral history:* Few interests outside of work prior to retirement Recent gradual decrease in activities with close family and friends	*Conduct a general reinforcer assessment:* What activities did Mr. and Mrs. Smith enjoy or find meaningful in the past? What skills did Mr. Smith have, and how can he still use them? Who is in their life now that would like to help?

mild congestive heart failure. Mrs. Jones was diagnosed with Alzheimer's disease 7 years ago. Mr. Jones is consulting you now because he is having increasing difficulty caring for his wife, who has become more and more confused. Her current MMSE score is 7/30. Mr. Jones says his wife has always worn the "pants in the family"; she had a "sharp tongue" with him and the children, but she has lately also started slapping and pinching him when he tries to help her with her personal care. He states that Mrs. Jones has stopped doing any housework, needs help with dressing, and often refuses to bathe. She is also getting up in the middle of the night, and he is worried that she may wander away from their house without his knowing about it. When Mr. Jones tries to talk to his wife about his concerns, she gets angry and tells him to "shut up" or "leave me alone."

A treatment for agitation has also been developed as part of the Seattle Protocols (Teri et al., 2003). Training using this approach would help Mr. Jones develop a greater appreciation of his wife's cognitive and functional limitations, teach him more effective ways of communicating with his wife, and point him toward supportive community resources. He would then be guided to identify the activators and consequences surrounding Mrs. Jones's agitated and aggressive behaviors using the A • B • Cs. Although Mrs. Jones is still living at home, her MMSE score is indicative of severe cognitive impairment, and it appears that she is no longer capable of complex verbal reasoning and discussion. This is the kind of client that the developers of need-based approaches had in mind: those with language difficulties, severe cognitive impairment, and a history of being somewhat disagreeable with other people even before the onset of dementia. Thus, in this case, it might also be useful to consider how the NDB model might be incorporated into your A • B • C analyses of Mrs. Jones's agitated behaviors.

NEED-DRIVEN THEORY: ACTIVATORS FOR AGITATION AND AGGRESSION

The NDB model considers individual characteristics, including stable or historical medical, cognitive, neurological, and psychosocial variables such as Mrs. Jones's lifelong short-tempered personality or her status as a matriarch within the household.[7] Individual background factors can be extremely helpful for understanding why some individuals, without apparent provocation, engage in behaviors that seem physically aggressive. For example, if the person with dementia has a history of boxing, martial arts, or military training, she may be unaware of her own strength and may be able to inflict serious harm quite unintentionally. If she grew up in a physically abusive household, lived

---

[7]According to the NDB model developed by Dr. Donna Algase and colleagues (1996), disruptive behaviors communicate basic needs or goals that people are unable to attain when their cognitive and functional impairments are severe. Treatment using the NDB approach does not follow a standardized protocol; rather, clinicians use the NDB model to develop individualized care plans for each situation. Background for the model is found in Algase et al. (1996) and Cohen-Mansfield (2000). Articles that can help the interested practitioner develop case-specific treatment interventions using this approach include Beck et al. (2002); Dettmore, Kolanowski, and Boustani (2009); Kolanowski, Litaker, and Buettner (2005); Whall et al. (2008); and Whall and Kolanowski (2004).

in communities with high levels of street and domestic violence, or has a history of anxiety, her deteriorating planning, foreseeing, and problem-solving skills, combined with visual disturbances, might make her more likely to strike out at others, even in the early stages of dementia. Most seemingly hostile behaviors from persons with dementia are defensive in nature, often aimed to reestablish the social standing once taken for granted by the person with dementia. Mrs. Jones has always liked being in charge of her family, and the dementia has not changed that. Generating awareness among caregivers that people with cognitive impairment are able to notice when they are treated with disrespect and are trying to maintain or recover their dignity often leads to improvements. Past behavior is always the best predictor of future behavior.

Consistent with activating comorbidities described in Chapter 5 of this book, the NDB model also discusses *proximal factors* and *need states* that can be activators for aggressive (i.e., self-protective) behavior. Proximal factors include Mr. Jones's attempts at personal care that precede his wife's slapping and pinching or aspects of the environment or daily routine that might be associated with her nocturnal wandering. Unmet physical or psychological needs might be further contributing to the observed behavior.[8] Within the NDB framework, needs communicated by self-protective or agitated behavior are commonly those arising from over- and understimulation, pain or discomfort, immobility, visual disturbances or hallucinations, depression, fatigue, and poor environmental design (e.g., insufficient lighting, inadequate outdoor access).

CONTEXTUAL MODEL: CONSIDER THE CONSEQUENCES

Background and proximal factors and need states would all be activators in Mrs. Jones's A • B • C functional analysis (see Exhibit 7.2). As such, they could be used to develop hypotheses about interventions that might reduce Mrs. Jones's agitation and aggression. Individualized assessment would assist Mr. Jones in recognizing early warning signs, so he could start deescalating Mrs. Jones's irritability before her behavior had gained momentum (e.g., by distraction and not contradicting her) and thus perhaps make crisis

---

[8]Although most primary "need states" in the NDB model are considered physiological (e.g., hunger, thirst, escape from pain, seeking comfort or stimulation), others such as modesty or respect may largely depend on verbally transmitted and socially reinforced rules of interpersonal conduct (Friman, Hayes, & Wilson, 1998). In our daily lives, sociocultural contingencies on following the rules of proper conduct (e.g., to earn delayed social rewards) mostly compete with the immediate fulfillment of physiological need. As dementia progresses, verbal capacity declines, and rules of conduct sometimes lose their hold, immediate needs may become much more salient and "override" social concerns, thereby generating the appearance of decreased predictability of a person's emotions and behaviors.

EXHIBIT 7.2
Use of NDB Constructs to Analyze Mrs. Jones's
Self-Protective Behavior and Nighttime Wandering

Activators	Behaviors
Proximal factors: • Intrusion of personal space Physiological need states: • Altered circadian rhythm? • Nighttime urinary urgency? Psychological need states: • Social standing • Autonomy • Safety Physical environment: • Bright hallway lighting at night? Social environment • Relationship with Mr. Jones	*Self-protective behaviors:* • Slapping. • Pinching. • Telling Mr. Jones to shut up and go away Dementia and confusion behaviors: • Wandering at night • Refusing to bathe

Broader psychosocial context/Gather a behavioral history:
Background factors:
• Severe dementia
• Decreased verbal skills
• Irritable premorbid personality
• Respected as matriarch

management medication treatment unnecessary.[9] The NDB model pays little attention to what happens after the target behavior and what might be maintaining Mrs. Jones's slapping, pinching, or telling Mr. Jones to "go away." Examining the consequences of dementia-related behaviors is important because it provides invaluable information about the function of the seemingly aggressive behavior. In this case, slapping, pinching, and yelling often succeeded in getting Mr. Jones to "shut up" and stop attempting the grooming activities his wife disliked. The behaviors thus inadvertently functioned to protect Mrs. Jones from incomprehensible interactions and discomfort. In addition, after each of these interactions, Mr. Jones then tended to speak in a soothing tone of voice, attending to Mrs. Jones in a very different and special

---

[9]In addition to the direct medication side effect risks described in Chapter 5, one little-considered risk of some psychotropic medications, particularly anxiolytics such as benzodiazepines, is that they can have addictive properties. There is always a possibility that medication that is given as needed or intermittently will be reinforcing, particularly if the person with dementia has a history of substance abuse. In this situation, a functional analysis will reveal whether the person's disruptive behavior functions as drug-seeking behavior. Note that from the contextual perspective, the behavior can be completely unintentional (i.e., the person with dementia engages in it but cannot describe its consequences). To learn about the well-established functions of drugs as antecedents or consequences, refer to McKim (2003) or Poling and Byrne (2000).

way. Mrs. Jones is subsequently more likely to try slapping or pinching again next time her husband is bothering her.[10]

THE STIGMA OF AGGRESSIVE BEHAVIOR

Analyzing consequences is also useful in the aftermath of self-protective behaviors because it reminds caregivers to resist automatically assuming that aggressive behavior is inevitable in a person with dementia. Consider Hattie's case.

> Hattie resided in a dementia care unit and had moderate to severe dementia. She could no longer express herself verbally or follow verbal instructions. Wheelchair bound and toothless because she refused to wear her dentures, Hattie spent her days propelling herself from resident to resident and kissing each person's hands. Although many residents removed their hands or shook Hattie off, her behavior was maintained by other residents and staff members who either tolerated the little kisses or kissed her back. Hattie's kissing, in general, did not pose a problem in the facility.
>
> When Hattie was hospitalized for pneumonia, her son called us to consult on his mom's "aggression" in the hospital. As it turned out, hospital staff—unfamiliar with Hattie—had interpreted her approaches as intentions to bite their hands. They called Hattie's son to inform him of the need for physical restraints. The son had not questioned the staff's report.

We see in this example that even close family members can be easily convinced that their loved one, who previously never hurt a fly, is capable of unprovoked attacks. It also illustrates how society stigmatizes people with cognitive impairment. Even professional providers sometimes speak of the "ABCs" of dementia as "aggression, behavior, and cognition." It bears repeating that dementia and aggressive behaviors do not inevitably go hand in hand. The popularized belief that dementia equals aggression tends to distort our judgments and interpretations, such that we might accept reports of aggression at face value and without further investigation. This fear of cognitively impaired individuals becomes further amplified if the person with dementia is an ambulatory, physically healthy, and tall man. Often, the stigma associated with dementia is so deeply engrained that even when the person is displaying out-of-the-ordinary and completely uncharacteristic

---

[10]Recent articles have expanded the NDB model to consider the larger chain of events surrounding dementia-related behaviors (Kovach, Noonan, Schlidt, & Wells, 2005; Woods, Rapp, & Beck, 2004), which in turn has also led to more elaborated conceptualizations of how such behaviors escalate and de-escalate over time.

behavior, we and family members tend to buy into the "unprovoked aggressive" interpretation of the behavior hook, line, and sinker. Instead, every report of aggressive action should be carefully investigated, and we would do so within the A • B • C format.

WANDERING AND CIRCADIAN RHYTHM DISTURBANCES IN DEMENTIA: JOANNE, PETER, HE LEN LEE, AND BOB

- Joanne walks continual laps with her walker in the hallway of the adult family home where she lives. When redirected to sit down, she does so readily, but as soon as the caregiver turns her back, she is heading back down the hall.
- Peter has been discovered outside of the memory care unit. He gained access to the gardens and jumped a 6-ft fence.
- He Len Lee was returned home by police officers after a Chinese restaurant owner called them. Mrs. Lee had visited the restaurant multiple times without eating there, and the restaurant owner was worried she was bothering the guests.
- Bob walked out of his home at 2 a.m. while the paid caregiver was watching late night TV. By the time his absence was noticed, he had walked several miles away in his pajamas and bare feet despite temperatures below freezing.

These four brief clinical examples demonstrate that when caregivers tell us their care recipient is "wandering," they often are referring to a range of different behaviors. For behaviors such as wandering that can have diverse topographies, the contextual model and A • B • C problem solving is really the ideal approach. For example, in the case of Joanne, from a contextual and behavioral point of view, the caregiver's kind attention to Joanne walking away may inadvertently reinforce her behavior (i.e., increase the likelihood that Joanne will walk again the next time she is left alone). This possibility could be tested by taking baseline A • B • C data and then suggesting to the caregiver that she attend to Joanne whenever she is doing something else other than walking. If Joanne's walking decreases in frequency over time during our intervention, yet increases again when the caregiver starts paying attention only when Joanne is walking away (i.e., on our return to baseline conditions), then our hypothesis would be borne out. However, wandering is also an example of the kind of behavior that is targeted by the PLST model, which emphasizes maximizing safety as part of its principles of care and recognizes the role that temporal patterns that occur in many dementia-related behaviors play. Thus, it might be helpful to consider how PLST could contribute to the behavioral analysis of the wandering cases described here.

PROGRESSIVELY LOWERED STRESS THRESHOLD: WANDERING AND CIRCADIAN RHYTHM DISTURBANCES TREATMENT

The PLST model postulates that persons can manage and adapt to stress in their daily lives up to a certain point or threshold above which their behavior becomes more anxious and dysfunctional. A dementing illness lowers this stress threshold, making it more difficult for those with dementia to cope with stress in their environment in an effective way. Six stressor categories are important for persons with dementia: fatigue, change (e.g., in routine, caregiver, environment), internal or external demands, multiple and competing stimuli, physical stress (e.g., illness, medication effects), and personal loss. Again, most of these stressors could be treated as activators in an A • B • C functional analysis. According to the PLST framework, manipulating one or more of the stressor categories can putatively reduce the stress experienced by the care recipient, which will reduce anxiety and onset of dysfunctional behavior. Caregivers are taught to identify peak periods of agitation so that stress-reducing activities can be planned to coincide with those times.

As with the NDB explanatory framework, treatment based on the PLST model does not follow a standardized protocol but is individualized based on principles of care that have been proposed to keep stress at a manageable level.[11] As such, treatment plans emphasize positive caregiver–care recipient interactions; creation of a simplified, secure, and pleasant environment; and care recipient activities and routines that help compensate for cognitive and functional losses. In the case of Joanne, the caregiver seems responsive to possible interpersonal or environmental stressors; she watches to see when Joanne gets up to walk and approaches her with unconditional positive regard, gently redirecting her back to her chair. She has not seen any temporal pattern to Joanne's wandering except that it only occurs during the day. The caregiver has not noticed Joanne exhibiting any other anxious or restless behaviors, nor is she wandering at night (so lack of sleep does not seem to be a factor).

---

[11]Although PLST can easily be used clinically in the absence of a treatment protocol, standardized protocols were used as part of the National Caregiver's Training Project (NCTP; Buckwalter, 1998). The NCTP study design and training protocol description are described in Gerdner, Hall, and Buckwalter (1996). For examples of other ways the PLST model has been applied to nursing care, and for detailed descriptions of the six principles of care, see Buckwalter et al (1999); Garand et al. (2002); Gerdner, Buckwalter, and Reed (2002); Lindsey and Buckwalter (2009); and Stolley, Reed, and Buckwalter (2002).

CONTEXTUAL MODEL: EXAMINING STRESSORS IN THE A • B • Cs

However, as is also the case with NDB, the PLST model does not tell us anything about the contingency relationship between a stressor, the target behavior, and its broader psychosocial context or consequences. Table 7.2 shows how Joanne's case might be regarded using the PLST concepts in combination with an A • B • C functional analysis. Emphasis is placed on identifying environmental activators that might be modified to enhance Joanne's safety and compensate for the loss of socialization she has experienced by moving out of her family home. The caregiver could implement a variety of meaningful activities to occupy Joanne and attend to her in the desired situation to see whether that reduces her wandering activity. The caregiver could

TABLE 7.2

Considering PLST Stressor Categories and Principles of Care
in Combination With the A • B • C Functional Analysis of Wandering

Activators	Behaviors	Consequences
Examine historical and proximal activators: External demands. Joanne's favorite chair is positioned so it faces the hallway. Physical stress. Joanne has arthritis that makes her knees hurt when she sits a long time. Loss. Joanne only walks when she is sitting by herself.	*Specify behavior of interest:* Joanne walks continual laps with her walker in the hallway of the adult family home where she lives. When redirected to sit down, she does so readily, but as soon as the caregiver turns her back, Joanne is heading back down the hall.	*Consider immediate consequences:* When Joanne starts walking, the caregiver stops her activities with other residents in the home and pays attention to Joanne. Joanne is complaining of shin pain.
Broader psychosocial context: Change. Joanne has recently moved to the AFH. Multiple or competing stimuli. When Joanne walks down the hall to her room, all the doors look the same.	*Gather a behavioral history:* Joanne has a large family and has always been surrounded by people and conversation.	*Conduct a general reinforcer assessment:* Are there activities that could keep Joanne pleasantly occupied?

Note. NDB = need-driven dementia-compromised behavior; PLST = progressively lowered stress threshold.

move Joanne's favorite chair so it looks out on a nearby schoolyard rather than down the empty hall. Maximizing Joanne's safety could include ensuring she always has her walker within reach so that she does not fall if she gets up, making sure Joanne takes her regular arthritis analgesic on the prescribed schedule to minimize her need to walk to relieve pain, and investigating whether Joanne needs to be wearing a different kind of walking shoe to reduce injury. The caregiver might also label the door to Joanne's room with a bright sign with her name so that if Joanne is seeking some quiet time resting in her room as she goes up and down the hall, she can find it. Implementing these kinds of changes and observing what happens as a result would guide the caregiver in deciding if the correct stressors or activators have been identified.

We can see from the example with Joanne that doing a full functional analysis adds precision to your understanding of the broader context in which her wandering developed. Neurodegenerative diseases undermine our physiological circadian rhythm mechanisms and stress responses, but often there are contributing historical, environmental, and psychosocial factors as well. As you read this, it might be helpful to brainstorm what activators and consequences might be operating in the cases of Peter, He Len Lee, and Bob. Do any of the clients have personal histories that have kept them physically active, and are they now trying to recreate that level of daily activity? Are there things in the physical environment that are waking people up at night, such as television noise and light? Is your client bored and seeking interaction with someone who will understand him or her? The different cells in the A • B • C table can help stimulate more ideas for you to consider in developing an individualized treatment plan.

WANDERING SAFETY

Regardless of the intervention model one follows, all individuals with dementia should wear a medical bracelet for safety's sake that identifies them and guarantees a return home (e.g., Alzheimer's Association "Safe Return" program). Installation of door alarms, sound monitors, or motion detector systems can alert a caregiver when a person tries to leave. Visual boundaries, such as a curtain hanging in front of a door, stop signs, or other cues, can prevent the person with dementia from trying to exit an area, although what will be effective will vary with each individual, depending on the level of cognitive function and the factors activating the person's intention to move. Many family caregivers consider locking the house doors and hiding the keys or installing locks out of reach of the person with dementia. However, these practices constitute safety hazards if the caregiver is ill, has suffered a debilitating accident, or is absent, because the person with dementia may not be able to work out how to leave the house in case of an emergency. A guide to home safety is available from the National Institute on Aging (*Home Safety for People with Alzheimer's Disease*, 2010).

ERRONEOUS BELIEFS AND ACCUSATORY BEHAVIOR IN DEMENTIA: MR. KOVAC

The management of erroneous beliefs and accusatory behavior in persons with dementia is one of the most challenging aspects of dementia care. Persons with dementia may accuse others of stealing their belongings, suspect ongoing activities behind their backs (e.g., affairs, schemes of exploitation), or feel that others are talking about or watching them. Family members often respond with fear and outrage and turn to their doctor for help when care recipients describe events that have not happened or when they accuse others of things they have not done. The most commonly prescribed treatment for such behaviors is an antipsychotic or anxiolytic medication (Madhusoodanan, Shah, Brenner, & Gupta, 2007). However, the U.S. Food and Drug Administration has not approved the use of medications for psychotic-like behaviors in persons with dementia, nor are medications very effective. As we have noted earlier, these medications are also associated with a whole host of other adverse side effects, including increased risk of mortality. Furthermore, our clinical observation has been that because these medications are highly sedating, they often impair general social function as well. Given that our clients' abilities to interpersonally communicate are already waning, do we want to take the risk of further negatively affecting their abilities to state their wants and needs, explain themselves, or engage in everyday conversation? Thus, as with the other mood and behavior changes we have been discussing, nonpharmacological options should always be considered the first-line interventions for erroneous beliefs and accusatory behaviors in older cognitively impaired individuals. All of the three models described in this chapter have been applied to persons with psychotic behaviors, but there are not yet good published data demonstrating their effectiveness, so the jury is still out on how best to treat them. In this section, we report our experience using the contextual A • B • C approach with clients who engage in accusatory behavior or act as if implausible events had happened, using Mr. Kovac as an example.

> Mr. Kovac is an 82-year-old widower living in an assisted living facility. He has called his son in the middle of the night on three occasions in the past month because he thought people were trying to break into his fourth floor apartment. He has also made several calls to 911 to report that money has been taken from his apartment. He blames the thefts on housekeeping staff and on his teenaged grandson who comes to visit with

his parents on Sundays after church. Mr. Kovac has stopped taking any meals in the common dining area because he says the other residents point and stare and talk about him. As a consequence, he is eating less and losing weight. He is also not sleeping well because of his fear of robbers, and he looks fatigued and disheveled. Yesterday he started an argument with the front desk volunteer. Mr. Kovac insisted his mailbox had been broken into and his Social Security check stolen, but the front-desk volunteer could not detect any evidence of damage to the mailbox lock.

CONTEXTUAL MODEL: ERRONEOUS BELIEFS AND ACCUSATORY BEHAVIORS

As with all of the cases described throughout this book, when working with clients who have erroneous beliefs and accusatory behaviors, we begin by trying to understand the behavior of our clients in the context in which it occurs. Neurodegenerative diseases are accompanied by a loss of the ability to describe or interpret reality. Nevertheless, our clients continue to give reasons, explain, and try to make sense of their world and to interpersonally connect with others by sharing their experiences. In the face of increasing cognitive impairment, it is not surprising that most erroneous beliefs involve theft and suspicion. In fact, what is more surprising is that more people with dementia do not develop such erroneous beliefs. We teach families that in the context of a progressive lack of reasoning ability, these inferences are normal responses to memory deficits and an inexplicably altered interpersonal context. Thus, the first step in caregiver training is to normalize the care recipient's inaccurate statements, given his or her condition, and to let caregivers know they have a choice in how to respond, even if their "buttons are being pushed." It is important to realize that our modern culture frowns heavily on inaccurate self-statements and fiction presented as fact. Thus, it is also normal for caregivers to have knee-jerk reactions of disappointment, anger, or even outrage to care recipients' delusional beliefs or accusations. Yet, even in the face of these reactions caregivers can work toward maintaining quality social interactions with the care recipient.

When persons with dementia present caregivers with facts or beliefs that are seemingly incorrect or erroneous, the caregiver or health care professional generally has several choices of how to respond. For example, two possibilities would be to gently (or forcefully) correct the inaccurate statement (reality orientation) or to ignore what the person has said and change the subject. Consider these two very different caregiver responses:

In the first scenario in Table 7.3, the caregiver skillfully accepts responsibility and offers a predictable and safe response that redirects the care recipient. (Such use of compassionate misinformation will be discussed in more

TABLE 7.3
Interactions Involving Erroneous Beliefs

Activators (care recipient utterance)	Caregiver behavior	Consequences (care recipient reaction)
1. "You have stolen my wallet."	"Oh, sorry; I took it to have its seam repaired. Let me see where I have it."	"Okay, next time, let me know so I don't have to search."
2. "You have stolen my wallet."	"No, I did not! *You* lost it again!"	"Yes, you have stolen it. I can see it in your face."

detail later.) As a result, the care recipient's accusation is fleeting. In contrast, the response by the second caregiver prompts the care recipient to reiterate his or her accusations. If we tracked the argument, the care recipient and caregiver of Example 2 might exchange the same accusations and responses back and forth multiple times, each insisting their viewpoint is "true."

From the contextual perspective, arguing with the care recipient not only draws more attention to the care recipient's accusation and prompts its repetition, it also raises the emotional stake and thereby creates the condition under which events are more likely to be remembered. It may well be the case that disputations and counterarguments reinforce (i.e., increase the frequency of) false beliefs. Moreover, the emotional upset related to interpersonal conflict may outlast the actual memory of what the conflict was about, such that caregivers begin to take on a vaguely negative emotional valence and become far more suspicious people, from the care recipient's perspective. For this reason, reality orientation is often contraindicated in the face of erroneous accusations. This general rule applies: If initial mild correction does not lead to a shift in the care recipient's reasoning, the caregiver may have to learn to let the care recipient be "right" regardless of content, quickly provide a plausible safety response, and not jeopardize the relationship (see Table 7.3, Example 1). We encourage a focus on the long-term outcome; it is often more important to stay in a good relationship with your client or loved one than to get the facts straight.

Other Functions of Erroneous Statements

When a care recipient's verbal abilities have declined significantly, erroneous statements may also contain implicit requests. For example, one of our clients repeatedly asked her in-home caregiving daughter, "Aren't my parents visiting this weekend?" The daughter was disturbed and did not know how to respond because her grandparents had passed away a long time ago. While brainstorming in the coaching session, the daughter remembered that the care recipient had cleaned the house from top to bottom before the grandparents' visits. When the daughter engaged her mother in more activity (including tasks that involved helping "clean" the house), the frequency with which the care recipient asked about her parents' visit dropped to zero. In other words, sometimes the historical consequences of a statement can inform its current purpose, in this case, the fact that the mother was bored (and perhaps did not think much of her daughter's housekeeping).

In other cases, the function of erroneous statements may be metaphorical. When clients without financial worries talk about fears of poverty, or an otherwise healthy person with dementia talks about illness and dying, they may be telling you about their losses and other age-related changes. Treatment for depression (i.e., activity engagement as described earlier) may change the person's verbalizations over time.

In still other cases, faulty statements and accusations may be the client's way of making sense of a world of memory impairment and shifting role identities or coping with inconceivable loss. Mr. Malloy, for example, was proud of his impeccable driving record and his driving skills. He used to please his wife by chauffeuring her. On receiving a letter from the Department of Motor Vehicles (DMV) for driver's testing, prompted by the neurologist's report, Mr. Malloy asked for help in maintaining his driving privileges. In our offices, Mr. and Mrs. Malloy signed releases for the exchange of information with the DMV. A day later, Mr. Malloy called the office and said he might have "mistakenly signed away" his driving privileges. Although we attempted a gentle correction of facts and invited Mr. Malloy to review the documents he had signed, Mr. Malloy said he was sure he signed the wrong papers and could not drive anymore. Thus, taking Mr. Malloy's concerns seriously, we apologized for the mix-up, and Mr. Malloy never drove again or inquired about his license. Instead, he maintained that at some point in time, he had signed the wrong document. Here, the erroneous statement functioned to preserve Mr. Malloy's dignity and his self-identity as an impeccable driver.

Erroneous Statements by Design: Compassionate Misinformation

Ironically, given the upset many caregivers experience over inaccurate statements made by care recipients, there comes a time for almost all caregivers when it is helpful to provide erroneous information to the person with dementia as a way of defusing potentially problematic situations. We were recently called to an assisted living facility to consult because a resident with dementia was walking into other residents' living areas and using their bathrooms to shower. We put up several signs pointing to the correct room ("Joe's bathroom"). When Joe complained that the signs offended him, we informed him that they served to orient the staff members. He accepted the explanation, and his showering in other residents' rooms decreased to zero.

As understanding and reasoning decline, there comes a point when the individual with dementia will not benefit from factually accurate information. For practitioners of dementia care, it is important to discern when this point has been reached. When is it more beneficial to the person to uphold factually inaccurate beliefs? When will the person benefit from compassionate misinformation that preserves dignity and self-identity, as in Mr. Malloy's driving story, rather than being told the truth? When will the truth overwhelm the person's coping skills and cause such rupture in relationships that it better be avoided?

Again, to advise the family, you will have to know the care recipient well. Questions such as the following can help you think about whether the person with dementia can understand and make beneficial use of factual information that has the potential to be upsetting.

- When you have informed the care recipient of your role, has he been able to recall it?
- Do your conversations with the care recipient "loop" around a narrow range of one or two topics, or is he or she still able to discuss a variety of topics with you?
- Does the care recipient utter mostly "stock phrases," remarks that could be applied to any situation, and eschew discussions of current happenings or feelings?
- Over the course of your meetings with the care recipients, have you repeated entire conversations, almost word-for-word?
- What has happened when you have provided factual information? Did the care recipient use it in subsequent conversation?

The decision to use compassionate misinformation should be a careful one. Using compassionate misinformation is contraindicated when the care recipient is still able to benefit from factual information. Note that the care recipient is as sensitive to feeling betrayed, deceived, lied to, and consequently disappointed and outraged as you are. When compassionate misinformation is used too early and without careful assessment, relationships may rupture and the care recipient may start distrusting a caregiver who seems a disloyal, manipulative conspirator. As a general rule, always gently orient the care recipient toward factual information first. Do not argue with the care recipient but simply suggest or inform. Then probe whether the care recipient has integrated the new factual information. If not, do not press on but use compassionate misinformation. Analogously, the family caregiver may engage in a similar assessment strategy, monitoring and documenting when informing and convincing do not work or when they threaten the relationship (A • B • C tracking sheets can be used for this purpose). If the presentation of factual information is contraindicated, collecting data on unworkable interactions shapes the caregiver's behavior toward a more compassionate approach. To use compassionate misinformation ethically, it must directly benefit and protect the person with dementia rather than the caregiver.

WHAT ABOUT ALTERNATIVE THERAPIES FOR DEMENTIA-RELATED MOOD AND BEHAVIOR CHANGES?

A variety of treatment approaches described in the dementia care literature are not part of the triad of evidence-based interventions we have been discussing. Should you or the client try aromatherapy, Snoezelen or multisensory therapy, music therapy, massage, touch, or dance therapies? What about validation therapy? There are also reminiscence and reality-orientation therapies. How does one decide what to do?

As a body of research, these alternative therapies have little evidence to support them. However, it should also be noted that from a contextual point of view, many alternative interventions and individualized activities such as music, art, dance, and reminiscence about the past may be perfectly appropriate consequence responses to a client's behavior or may serve as ways to address client needs or to lower stress in their environments. For example, after we have conducted an assessment of the A • B • Cs, including the person's history and preferences, we may find out he used to enjoy singing in a choir. Joining a small singing group or entering a music program to inspire and rekindle the old preferences then makes sense. You may think to yourself, "Oh, this is nothing but music therapy." For us, however, what counts is the rationale for trying this particular strategy with this particular person, as justified by the A • B • C assessment.

A functional analysis places emphasis on an ongoing monitoring of outcome and a return to the drawing board, if necessary. Thus, from the contextual model perspective, we value how the intervention fits that particular person with his or her history and current circumstances, and how its implementation plays out in the person's life. Connecting with historically important activities and memories not only provides a rich source of positive activators and reinforcing consequences to influence behavior patterns, they also bring an overall richness and quality to the lives of both care recipient and caregiver. This allows both caregiver and care recipient to enjoy the journey a bit more, which is the subject of our next chapter.

8

ENJOY SHARING THE JOURNEY: SUPPORTING A GOOD QUALITY OF LIFE

This brings us to the last element of the dementia DANCE for providers: helping clients and caregivers sustain a good quality of life. As we have emphasized throughout this book, dementia is a very personal disease. You, the health care provider, have come to know your clients' current circumstances, their histories, dreams, and values. You have helped to rule out and treat any comorbidities that add to the burden of a dementing illness. You have worked to strengthen the caregiving relationship and assisted in developing behavioral change plans that are tailored to each unique dyadic situation. Now, the real work lies ahead: encouraging your clients and caregivers, day-by-day, to continue living life to its fullest.

When we give clients a new diagnosis of dementia, we always remind them that they are the same person today as they were yesterday before receiving this news. Life down the line is going to change, to be sure, but patients with Alzheimer's are not the only people who experience change and loss. Every chronic illness, and for most of us aging itself, brings about life adjustments that we would not choose to experience. At the same time, most of us also find that these unwanted "opportunities" often have blessings embedded in them as well as pain. It is not unusual for health professionals to see their dementia clients and caregivers periodically over many years' duration and to have the privilege of helping them negotiate many transitions as dementia progresses. At each point along the way, it is important to remind them that love, laughter, friendship, and personal meaning are also still part of their life story.

THE #1 TOOL FOR QUALITY OF LIFE: ENGAGEMENT IN MEANINGFUL ACTIVITIES

Referrals to health care providers are often made for behaviors such as wandering, anger and agitation, or accusatory behavior and erroneous beliefs. The labeling of these behaviors as "problems" is to some extent a matter of perspective. The experimental psychology literature shows that organisms prefer to walk away from or avoid unpleasant situations (Ulrich & Azrin, 1962). If there is no opportunity for escape, organisms engage in self-protective, "aggressive" behavior. In other words, from the contextual standpoint, many behavioral and affective changes in persons with dementia are "normal" responses to a life of decreasing personal autonomy and an increasingly restricted lifestyle.

In addition, persons with dementia are often aware of their increasing difficulties and are embarrassed about them. They start to avoid daily activities and routines that they anticipate could lead to social disapproval or public humiliation. As noted in the previous chapter, the result can be a spiral of depression and further social withdrawal that is hard to break. Fortunately, treatment of depression through increased access to individualized meaningful activities and pleasant social interactions is one of the most effective and generalizable interventions available in dementia care.

What Is Meaningful Activity?

Meaningful activity is anything a person does that brings joy or a sense of purpose or fulfillment. Clients and caregivers usually can identify many things that they used to enjoy doing but no longer can because of the care recipient's dementia symptoms. Traveling to exotic places; attending movies and plays; participating in bridge teams, cooking classes, and book clubs; deer hunting; bowling; crocheting; and even going to large family holiday dinners become too much to handle. Thus, the challenge for practitioners and family members alike lies in discovering and implementing events that are meaningful and still doable for the person with dementia, however impaired he or she may be. It is important to keep in mind that activity for activity's sake does not work. As Robert Davis (1989) so aptly noted, "I have the right [to refuse] any activity or entertainment that I do not perceive as entertaining" (p. 102).

Along these same lines, one of our clients dryly noted, "I will not participate in forced fun." To find activities that fit the lives of individuals with dementia, we have to think outside the box, to move beyond daytime TV, bingo, and other stereotypical "pleasant" activities for adults 60 years and older and find creative, simplified variants of activities on a continuum with what the person would have done in the past, even if it was effortful.

Meaningful activities must also have continuity with the person's values. For example, many in the post-World War II generation placed a high value on the importance of service to family and community. Cognitively impaired individuals can still continue to "serve" their families and communities if we allow them to assist with tasks that do not necessarily require performance precision; washing windows, setting tables, making beds, rinsing dishes, folding towels, sweeping floors, sorting magazines, feeding or brushing pets, "volunteering" at the adult day center, and accompanying staff on their rounds at the nursing home are all examples of service activities that can give a person a continued sense of accomplishment and usefulness.

Identifying Meaningful Activities

Looking through family picture albums and asking clients to reminisce, either alone or with their family or friends, about the past can give many clues as to what categories of meaningful or valued activities would be good to explore in the present.[1] Was the person an avid hobbyist? If she no longer can crochet, does she still enjoy handling skeins of yarn? If he no longer can build furniture, would he still enjoy sanding an old end table? Artisans of all sorts often continue to enjoy practicing a simplified version of their craft or looking at samples of their work. Sorting through CD boxes or old record albums or listening to a preferred style of music can be extremely pleasurable to people who played music, attended concerts, or loved to sing and dance. Insatiable readers often find deep satisfaction reading or looking through old letters or at some of the many beautiful children's books that are available in libraries today. Outdoor enthusiasts may enjoy sitting at a window or on the porch admiring their birdbath and garden or sitting on a park bench watching children play on

---

[1]For people looking for ideas for pleasant activities for care recipients, Dowling's (1995) classic book offers 12 chapters with different categories of activities, such as humor, exercise, art, and pets, to name a few examples. Teri and Logsdon (1991) have also developed a Pleasant Events Schedule for persons with dementia. Caregivers can rate simple pleasant activities both in terms of the frequency with which they have occurred in the past month and how enjoyable the care recipient found each activity in the past and finds it now. This rating system provides a good way of thinking about activities not on any list as well; if an activity that has not been done in a while brings the care recipient pleasure, it is worth trying it again now. Conversely, if the activity is something the care recipient does every day but has never enjoyed (e.g., sitting on a couch watching TV), then it may not be a meaningful activity now, even if it does provide a useful function for the caregiver by occupying the care recipient's time.

the swing sets. Brainstorming about pleasant valued activities heavily over-laps with our discussion in Chapter 6 about preserving role relationships. The more our clients with dementia are viewed as persons of worth whose prefer-ences and opinions still matter, as men and women who have something to offer the world, the better will be their quality of life.

Increasingly, communities as well as families are recognizing the value of supporting continued involvement by persons with dementia in life-enriching programs. The "Meet Me at MoMA" Alzheimer's Project of the Museum of Modern Art in New York, for example, began in 2006 to involve individuals with dementia and their caregivers in the creation and discussion of art (Rosenberg, 2009). In the true spirit of *de gustibus non est disputandum* (taste is not a matter of discussion), each person is entitled to his or her eval-uation and impression and to his or her creation. The program does commu-nity outreach and has branched out to smaller cities (e.g., http://www.momentsofmemory.org). In the greater Washington, DC, area, Lolo Sarnoff's "Arts for the Aging" Project (http://www.lolosarnoff.com/afta.html) has for the past 3 decades fulfilled a similar purpose of restoring self-esteem and well-being and diminishing frustration. Such programs allow those with dementia who may know nothing about art to voice preferences and express reactions in a context where "right" or "wrong" are meaningless. What matters most is that each person's voice, in all its individuality, is heard.

CHALLENGES TO MEANINGFUL ACTIVITIES

Research over the past decade has shown that even when persons with dementia consider their own quality of life to be quite good, caregivers tend to rate their care recipients' quality of life much lower.[2] In line with our dis-cussion of reinforcement erosion in Chapter 6, caregivers seem to focus more on what they and their loved ones have lost rather than on what they still have and are capable of. At the beginning of treatment, the glass is frequently half-empty. This mind-set can make it challenging for caregivers to think cre-atively about activities that the care recipient might still be able to partici-pate in and enjoy. An adult daughter never considers offering a coloring book to her dignified artistic mother with dementia until Mom begins taking the grandchildren's books and crayons and using them herself. In the documen-tary *Complaints of a Dutiful Daughter* (1994), filmmaker Deborah Hoffman described her initial shock over her college-educated and sophisticated

---

[2]Information on the Quality of Life in Alzheimer's Disease rating scale and its correlates with caregiver and care recipient variables can be found in Logsdon, Gibbons, McCurry, and Teri (1999, 2002).

mother's enjoyment of Ed McMahon's TV program *Star Search:* "This is not my mother. This is beneath her!" This difficulty identifying meaningful activities is increased when care recipients are depressed and verbalizing feelings of worthlessness and a general unwillingness to do anything. Nevertheless, it is important to try. Depression in persons with dementia is a stronger predictor of low quality of life ratings by both caregivers and care recipients than either cognitive and functional impairment or caregiver burden. In many cases, the single most effective thing caregivers can do to improve their own and their care recipient's situation is to help the person with dementia stay engaged in pleasurable and personally meaningful life activities.

The biggest problem with increasing pleasant and meaningful activities is that it relies heavily on caregivers' energy, inclination, and availability. Can the caregiver drive the person with dementia to activities? Does he have the skills to investigate and work with community agencies to find a good activity match for the care recipient? Is she willing to tolerate the discomfort of exposing the care recipient to new and unfamiliar situations or to activities that the caregiver (but perhaps not the care recipient) may consider "silly" or "demeaning"? Is he juggling a job and parenthood as well as supervising the care of a mother with dementia? Is she physically ill or exhausted? In long-term care settings, insufficient staffing and turnover can make it difficult to develop individualized programming for each resident. For all these reasons, social withdrawal and activity restriction are not usually at the top of the list of pressing concerns for family and professional caregivers. Thus, it is wise for the health care professional to anticipate that there will be setbacks in caregivers' initiation and follow-through with activity planning. You can play an important role by helping caregivers and institutions identify potential obstacles to activities and find strategies for overcoming barriers if they arise.

SIMPLE PLEASURES COUNT

One useful place to start with caregivers who are already stretched thin with worry and responsibility is to help them come to understand that pleasant and meaningful activities do not necessarily have to involve a lot of additional work, cost, and time. Dr. Linda Teri at the University of Washington developed a training program for direct care staff working in assisted living facilities with cognitively impaired residents.[3] The program teaches staff that

---

[3]The Staff Training in Assisted Living Residences program is described in a series of articles by Teri et al. (Teri, Huda, et al., 2005; Teri et al., 2009, 2010).

"every interaction can be a pleasant event" and "pleasant events are everyone's job." The consequences of such an approach can be dramatic. One of our clients was wheelchair bound and living in an adult family (board and care) home. We were called in because the resident was sleeping all day and staying up all night. In less than a month, the resident's sleep–wake pattern was restored to normal by a simple change instituted in the home: Every time a daytime caregiver would walk by, he or she would touch the resident in a gentle way, bend down and smile, look in his eyes, and speak to him using his name. As a result of these brief but repeated personal contacts, the resident started staying awake for longer and longer periods during the day. When he was awake, he was looking around more and seemed more engaged with what was going on in the home. The staff reported a growing fondness for this gentleman, who, up to that point, had been almost invisible to day staff and mostly a bother to those working nights. The man's apparent quality of life was greatly enhanced by this seemingly tiny change, and to all appearances, his professional caregivers were happier too. Little things can make a big difference even to those who are unable to describe how they feel, what they need, or what happened to them today, during the last hour, or in the last 5 minutes.

For family caregivers, another simple but powerful tool is helping them discover activities that facilitate the transition to a world where "being with each other" is more important than knowing facts or how to get things done. Persons who have lived together or been friends a long time are accustomed to a certain style of interaction and ways of being in one another's company that do not always work well once one of the parties has dementia. For example, many of us connect to each other by talking, informing, and exchanging facts. One of our clients and her daughter greatly enjoyed playing *Jeopardy* and other trivia games, competing for the best and fastest answers. Even outside of game playing, much of their friendly banter tended toward a question and answer style that included few periods of silence. With Mom's increasing word-finding and naming difficulties, these trivia games and lively conversations became too demanding. To the daughter, the mother's prolonged silences—when Mom could not think of anything to bring up or drew blanks—felt like "silent treatment," hurtful and rejecting. We suggested that together they attend a gentle yoga and meditation class for seniors as a way of helping both mother and daughter experience periods of prolonged silence in a nonthreatening context. Mom and daughter enjoyed the practice, and even after they stopped attending the class, they continued to use the class sounds and music at home to create the same friendly and relaxed environment. From an A • B • C perspective, the intervention established activators or a context in which being with each other in silence (B) was not only tolerated but also welcomed (C).

LOOKING FOR SAFETY BUBBLES

Safety bubbles is a term we use to describe those situations or contexts in which a care recipient's inability to render factual information is completely irrelevant. Safety bubbles are those times and places where it is impossible at first glance to tell the difference between someone with dementia and everyone else. What freedom for the cognitively impaired individual! What relief to be somewhere that you have no concerns about "right" and "wrong," "accurate" or "incorrect," or "true" and "false." A colleague recently told us about placing his cognitively impaired father in a dementia care unit. At home, Dad had been irritable, angry, and even unpredictably physically assaultive, despite all best efforts to provide the best combined medication and nonpharmacological care. Once Dad was in the new setting, however, he settled down. The colleague observed that the biggest difference seemed to be that his dad was "no longer at home, where we all expected him to act normal. In a place where nobody acts normal, the pressure is off."

You do not have to move to a nursing home, however, to find a safety bubble. Many communities such as adult day centers or programs such as "Meet Me at MoMA" are aiming for the same experience. These and similar programs can help reestablish, maintain, or build caregiver–care recipient relationships in a low-pressure setting. Imagining safety bubbles also helps one think more broadly and imaginatively about possibilities for pleasant and meaningful events. Does the activity help the person maintain feelings of dignity and self-respect? Is the situation devoid of pressure to remember people, places, or events? Is it an opportunity for strengths rather than deficits? Is it free of over-stimulating or overwhelming demands? An ancient matriarch half-dozing in a comfortable chair in the middle of a holiday gathering with family stopping by every few minutes to give her a kiss and rub sweet-smelling hand cream into her gnarled but oh-so-soft hands is in the ultimate safety bubble. She is valued without any performance demands. Everyone loves her; everyone knows that they are there because of her, whether she recognizes them or not. In contrast, a mildly impaired, recently retired businesswoman—also the matriarch of her family—might experience the same situation as irritating and demeaning. Her safety bubble would be one in which she could actively participate, possibly guiding and caring for others. Again, we must always tailor our interventions to the unique person.

COMPASSIONATE MISINFORMATION IN THE SAFETY BUBBLE

In Chapter 7, we used the term *compassionate misinformation* to refer to those times when we either allow the person with dementia to hold a belief that is not true or we offer an explanation that is not factually accurate in the service of defusing potentially problematic situations. The function of compassionate information in the safety bubble is to help a person maintain their role identity and support interpersonal connections. A husband is not lying when he chooses not to correct his wife as she tells her neighbor about sitting next to President Obama on a recent subway ride. Rather, the husband is allowing his wife to enjoy the pleasure she derives from telling people about an event that was interesting and made her feel good, even if it is an event that did not actually happen. Such storytelling inaccuracies or confabulations about recent and remote past events are common in persons with dementia, and they often serve to help individuals actively contribute to a social situation.

Even more common are those instances in which the caregiver is invited to hear the same story (accurate or not) over and over and over again. If the story is one that provides pleasure to the storyteller, then what is to be gained by saying, "Dad, you already told me that one"? For Dad, who does not remember telling you that one 10 minutes ago, it is a brand new story to be experienced with the same gusto it had every time previously. Compassionate misinformation can also be a way of protecting the care recipient from truths that are painful and best forgotten. It is a kindness to not correct Mom when she tells everyone at the nursing home that her son will be coming to visit next month, even though you know the son died a decade ago. Her story also allows you an opportunity to ask about other pleasurable memories of the son: "Tell me what he is like," "Let us look at his pictures together." Such reminiscences help the person with dementia connect their increasingly fragmented past and present, practice telling stories, and connect with another human being, even if the shared memories were never actual events.

SUPPORTING CAREGIVER QUALITY OF LIFE

Helping care recipients engage in pleasant and meaningful activities and creating safety bubbles not only help the person with dementia, but these activities also improve the caregiver's quality of life. When care recipients are happier, less depressed and less anxious, feeling less threatened or less worthless, their increased well-being is a bonus for those who live with and love them. However, caregivers also have their own separate needs for assistance and quality of life support that are independent from those of the person with dementia. Caregivers are analogous to flight attendants on a long transatlantic flight. The flight may be bumpy or smooth; at any point in time there may a lull in activity or an unexpected emergency may erupt. The passengers may be cheerful or cranky, compliant or demanding, asleep or pacing the aisle. Unlike the passengers, who are mostly just along for the ride, making the best of their situation, the flight attendants are continually busy trying to ensure that the trip is as comfortable, safe, and pleasant as possible. To do this job well, the attendants need to make sure that they are rested, physically healthy, and mentally alert. It is worth noting that happier caregivers make for happier care recipients too, not just vice versa. Individuals with dementia can sense when all is not well with the people around them. If either a caregiver or you, the health care provider, becomes sick and burned out, you increase the likelihood that the care recipient will manifest his or her concerns with behaviors that will only make your situation more difficult.

Caregiver Health

There is a large body of literature indicating that caregivers are at increased risk of adverse health problems.[4] Caregivers self-rate their health more poorly than noncaregivers and are more likely to get insufficient rest, to neglect taking prescription medications, and to not take sufficient time to recover from illnesses when they occur. They have higher levels of stress hormones, lower levels of antibody responses, greater body mass index, and increased rates of hypertension, cardiovascular disease, and elevated cholesterol and insulin levels. These physiological side effects of caregiving are greatest when caring for individuals with pronounced affective and behavioral changes, and they can persist long after active caregiving ends.[5]

Thus, the importance of helping caregivers adopt healthier lifestyles cannot be overstated. Health care professionals should inquire into caregivers' habits and routines: Do you smoke? Do you drink alcohol, and if so, how often, in what quantity, and at what time(s) of day? Are you gaining or losing weight? When was the last time you saw your physician for a checkup? Have you told your doctor about any changes in your health or any difficulties in following his or her treatment recommendations, such as keeping to a certain diet? How much sleep do you get on average? In particular, you should ask caregivers about their exercise habits. Although regular physical activity

---

[4]There are a number of pertinent reviews and articles describing the health consequences of caregiving (e.g., Burton, Newsom, Schulz, Hirsch, & German, 1997; de Vugt et al., 2003; Esterling, Kiecolt-Glaser, Bodnar, & Glaser, 1994; Gouin, Hantsoo, & Kiecolt-Glaser, 2008; Schulz & Martire, 2004; Schultz, O'Brien, Bookwala, & Fleissner, 1995; Schulz & Sherwood, 2008; Vitaliano, Zhang, & Scanlan, 2003). There is also a growing body of research examining the role of exercise in caregiver health (e.g., Janevic & Connell, 2004; King, Baumann, O'Sullivan, Wilcox, & Castro, 2002).

[5]Research indicates that a sizable percentage of caregivers do not show improvement in their emotional functioning after active caregiving ends but continue to have stable or even increased symptoms of emotional distress and depression for years afterward (Aneshensel, Botticello, & Yamamoto-Mitani, 2004; Robinson-Whelen, Tada, MacCallum, McGuire, & Kiecolt-Glaser, 2001). The greater the role overload during the active caregiving period, the greater the likelihood of continued emotional distress after caregiving ends. This speaks to the importance of getting caregivers effective help in dealing with their situation as early in the process as possible.

is not a "magic bullet" for caregiver stress and strain, it does lower risk of developing many common disabling age-related illnesses and also may provide an important avenue for social interactions outside the home. However, to succeed in a regular exercise program, caregivers not only need someone to stay with the care-recipient but also need substantial encouragement, in some sense "permission" from health care providers, family members, and friends.

Caregiver Burnout

Unfortunately, it is still rare for caregivers to seek out the assistance of health care professionals for themselves when dementia is first diagnosed. Many caregivers are for years a "one-person-show," progressively restricting their activities exclusively to caregiving until they suddenly reach the end of their rope. Under these strained circumstances, your emphasis on shared meaningful events—even if you have determined them to be essential to the well-being of the care recipient and the caregiver—will fall on barren soil. Although caregivers who come to you early on learn to live well with dementia, caregivers arriving at your door after years of isolation are focused on merely surviving rather than living well. They might be considering abandoning their loved ones on the steps of the closest emergency room. They might fantasize about escape, something one of our colleagues called "white-line-fever": following that white highway divider line toward the horizon. When you ask these caregivers, "What would you like to have happen?" they might not be able to state their wants or needs anymore because they have not considered them in years. Their lives might have been an accumulation of "ought-tos" and "musts." Here, a possible path in the journey involves a slow rebuilding of the caregiver's life to the point at which the caregiver will be able to engage in self-care and enjoy the care recipient's presence again.

Working with caregivers who present with burnout—hopelessness, depression, resentment, and exhaustion—requires a careful examination of the situation and the implementation of respite services as quickly as possible. If a caregiver seems reluctant to act or agrees to and then does not follow through with a respite plan, it is worthwhile exploring the following issues, regardless of the number of years that the caregiver has been providing care:

- Has the caregiver accepted the care recipient's diagnosis?
- Does the caregiver understand the relationship between the dementia syndrome and the caregiving challenges he or she has been experiencing?
- Are there sociocultural rules that prevent the caregiver from applying your advice?

- Is the caregiver an accurate reporter of circumstances, and would a home visit be helpful in understanding the caregiver's and care recipient's actual situation?
- Is the caregiver an accurate reporter of his or her own needs, or does he or she tend to minimize concerns rather than "be a bother" or appear weak or incompetent?
- Does the caregiver have the interpersonal skills to interact with doctors, agencies, and other providers successfully?
- Does the caregiver have a history of conflict with the care recipient that makes the current situation appear more "normal" than it actually is?
- Is the caregiver an active problem-solver or prone to avoid conflict with wishful thinking or escape through use of mood-altering substances?
- Does the caregiver feel comfortable asking family and friends for help, or has he or she always been the "lone ranger" who relied on him- or herself to get things done?
- Does the caregiver understand the reciprocal relationship of lifestyle and mood? Does he or she have a self-care repertoire involving proper nutrition, hydration, sleep, exercise, medical and dental care, and so forth?

Depending on the answers to these questions, your own professional background, and the resources you have available in your practice, you might decide to implement evidence-based social skills training, mindfulness, or depression protocols. We often refer to other providers in the community when skills deficits are severe, mental health problems have been chronic, or the caregiver is willing to address her substance use in therapy. Regardless of whether we collaborate with other providers or use in-house resources to build skills, helping caregivers to overcome barriers to their own quality of life is one of the most rewarding aspects of our work.

When Long-Term Care Is the Best Answer

For most caregivers, the day eventually comes when moving the care recipient into residential care outside the family home is the best solution for all parties concerned. Some caregivers ruminate about this day for years in advance, wondering, "How will I know when it is time?" The answer to that question, like every other aspect of good dementia care, is highly individualized. For some caregivers, residential care is needed once a care recipient starts having trouble with their basic activities of daily living: eating with utensils, walking without falls, or continence of urine or bowel. Other caregivers do not feel needed anymore once the care recipient no longer recognizes them or the familiar surroundings and repeatedly asks to go home or calls the caregiver by a different name. Particularly when persons are difficult to distract or redirect (and might have a related history of abuse by or mistrust of others), not knowing where they are or who is with them can lead to intractable agitation, restlessness, attempts to escape, or other physically self-protective behaviors.

In yet other cases, the caregiver's own physical health, emotional exhaustion, or competing life demands will necessitate arranging a move before the care recipient has experienced severe cognitive decline. Some individuals with dementia are able to plan for their move and participate in the selection of the long-term care setting. They can visit facilities with you, friends, or family members and judge whether they could fathom living in the setting, even if they do not have specific memories of the visits after the fact. Moving becomes a collaborative and agreeable venture, and all of the care recipient's concerns are validated and taken into account. Other times, the care recipient seems cognizant enough to understand what is happening but is not in agreement that moving is a good idea. Not safe at home alone and open to exploitation and accidents, such individuals need to move, but discussing the pros and cons of what a move might look like is highly fear inducing and overwhelming. The care recipient may refuse to talk about a move, cry and beg the caregiver to delay, attempt to run away, rant and rave or even assault people around them, or threaten suicide. In these cases, the care recipient's memory may be largely intact, yet reasoning and planning skills may be on the wane. Such cases are the most agonizing for caregivers who may spend months to years postponing a needed decision or second-guessing the one they made, even when the outcome for the care recipient has been positive.

It is important to work with caregivers to see that in most cases, everyone's reaction to this most difficult of decisions is comprehensible, given the current circumstances, dementia severity, and the caregiver and care recipient's personal histories of coping with distress. Logical reasoning with the care recipient to convince him that this is "for his own good" (a phrase that is open to multiple interpretations) is virtually never useful. One of our most frequent uses of compassionate misinformation is in strategizing with families to prepare an individual for respite care or residential placement. Consider the following examples:

- Genevieve's favorite narrative was how she came to know her now deceased husband and how much they loved each other during their 60-plus-year marriage. She happily recalled how she and her husband had first owned a small condominium during their early years. When the family explained to her that her husband had left her a condominium to care for her after his death, she gladly moved to the room of the specialized dementia care unit. Once there, she continued to tell staff how much her husband loved her and how he had bought the "condo" for her.

- After his wife died, Geoffrey refused to get out of bed for weeks at a time. Concerns about social withdrawal and isolation, in combination with cognitive decline related to Alzheimer's disease, prompted the family to consider a specialized dementia care unit. Geoffrey had a history of hotel management, and he and his wife had been enthusiastic travelers. Consequently, the family informed the care recipient he would move to a new hotel in town to "try it." Geoffrey moved into the "hotel" with only a few belongings. Over time, the family brought more of his personal belongings. Geoffrey told his family members he was in a "six-star hotel" and never asked about returning home.

MOVING ON TO THE NEXT STAGE

As seen in the these two examples, a move into residential care is often good for the care recipient, not the disaster that both the person with dementia and the caregiver had anticipated. One still-working caregiver told us that he was distressed after moving his wife into a specialized dementia care unit and tried to visit her for many hours every day, despite the considerable strain that was placing on his job and finances. One day he asked his wife how she coped when she was alone without him. She told her husband that she didn't miss him at all: "You were always working late and traveling for the company. I'm used to keeping busy when I'm by myself." Indeed, staff confirmed that when the husband was absent, his wife strolled the halls, emptied and repacked her dresser drawers, and seemed fairly content. This information allowed the caregiver to give himself permission to move to a less frequent visitation schedule that allowed him to enjoy the time he had with his wife to a greater degree. We often tell caregivers that a successful transition is one in which caregivers visit and their loved ones do not have time for them because they are engaged in facility-organized or incidental activities (e.g., helping water the courtyard shrubs).

Some caregivers find the transition into a life without the daily responsibilities of care more difficult. Unlike the death of a spouse or parent, the care recipient is still living, and the caregiver still has some level of emotional connectedness and ultimate responsibility for the oversight of the person's care. Changing routines, breaking habits, and establishing new lifestyle patterns are all hard. In addition, moving a person requires skillful interactions with administrators, nurses, and other facility staff. Family caregivers must learn to distinguish between when their intervention and advocacy is needed, and when the care recipient's report can be acknowledged without further follow-up. For example, the care recipient might be awakened and bothered by screaming in the facility and might complain to the caregiver. In this case, an investigation by the caregiver would reveal that one resident briefly screams during the nightly shift change, and an intervention on her behalf could solve the problem for both residents. In another case, a caregiver's spouse may report that he "had to set the workers straight last night." This statement may function to maintain the person's identity because he was a foreman, and may not need investigation or follow-up. Finding the balance between problem-focused coping and acceptance of a loved one's changing reality as dementia progresses is difficult. We often tell caregivers we would like them to build "muscles" that provide the strength for the new road ahead. These muscles might be sore and fatigued on some days from the newness of the experience, but over time, they will make the journey easier and the step lighter.

Thinking of this life transition as a kind of exercise or journey for which caregivers have to train makes the change seem somehow more manageable. This can be a good time to teach caregivers systematic relaxation or mindfulness exercises, to explore long-neglected opportunities for intellectual stimulation (e.g., signing up for a course, taking up an old hobby), to help them connect with social communities that may have been neglected, or even do a leisurely yet thorough "spring cleaning" of the house and yard. It is also a good time to revisit the discussion about maintaining healthy habits when things are difficult. In the absence of a care recipient to look after, some caregivers lose the motivation to eat regular meals; some may start drinking more heavily because time feels so heavy on their hands; still others may fall into irregular sleep–wake patterns that initially appear positive ("I can finally sleep in all I want!") but can be quite maladaptive in the long run.

Note that when working with caregivers at this transition phase, their thoughts and feelings must always be acknowledged. We do not dispute their personal experience or try to convince them to see the "bright side of life" or to feel differently. Caregivers value the role they are playing in the life of the individual who has dementia, whether out of obligation, duty, love, or reciprocity. They are trying their best, with the tools they have available. We do encourage caregivers to reflect on their values, however, and to see where this latest stage of moving on to separate living fits in their caregiving story.

Caring does not end when the person with dementia moves into a facility. Grief over not sleeping with a beloved at night can mingle with pride for having cared for him or her so long and with laughter over some of the times shared long ago. For the health care professional who may have worked for many years with the family living with dementia, this is an opportunity to also share one's own stories and memories with the caregiver and to reflect on what has been learned from the family's struggle and example. It can be a profound and healing aspect of your professional relationship and one that you both will remember for many years yet to come.

III

CONCLUSION

9

GOING THE DISTANCE: YOUR LONG-TERM ROLE

It is no exaggeration to say that clinicians who work with persons with dementia are among the most unselfish, caring, and committed health care professionals to be found. If you have read this book, chances are that you are one of them! Throughout this book, we have offered multiple examples and tools to help you work even more effectively with your clients, their caregivers, and your colleagues who collaborate in their care. Dementia care, however, can be intense. The behavioral and affective changes experienced by individuals with dementia and their families touch the core of human existence. As dementia clients and their families grapple with changing identities, visions for the future, helplessness, and fear of infirmity and death, you walk along the path with them. Indeed, your role as health care professionals is to be a steady compass that will enable your clients to follow their path (i.e., respond to the dementia's challenges in a way that is consistent with their values) even when it is dark and the road is unfamiliar. In this final chapter, we invite you to consider what you need to do to ensure that you also do not lose yourself along the way.

BUILDING DEEP CONNECTIONS IN THE MOMENT

We have found three things that have helped us and the trainees we work with to stay inspired, energized, and hopeful. The first is the realization that effective dementia care creates opportunities for persons with dementia and their families to engage with each other in positive ways and experience connectedness and joy, regardless of level of cognitive impairment. To be fully human is to be in relationship with other people. The underlying premise of this book is that persons with dementia are fully human in this most essential way. As health care professionals, we can help our clients with dementia and their caregivers enhance and rekindle their relationships and maintain a high quality of life in the presence of progressive cognitive decline. At the same time, sharing these opportunities for connectedness and joy with your clients can deepen your own sense of life purpose and meaning.

What is it about dementia care that makes it so uniquely positioned to help health professionals connect and engage with their clients? We think it is because readiness to develop a thorough understanding of our clients is a prerequisite for the job. People who are losing their ability to complete stepwise tasks or remember recent events also lose familiar social strengths and relationships and often become afraid. When someone is losing his or her memory and most treasured skills in seemingly unpredictable and incomprehensible ways, the health care provider can be a human lifeline offering understanding and hope. Providers working with persons with dementia are not only sources of information and skills training but they are also people to whom their clients can turn for deeper reassurance and support, often for years to come.

There is a deep and important reassurance and support that comes from simply being with another person, even after language and reasoning fail. Our expert language skills count for little when interacting with a person with advanced dementia. Instead, like new parents, we go back to the basics: taking time to learn about the person's history and preferences, closely observing his or her behavior to anticipate needs, and using physical cues, such as smiles, eye contact, and tone of voice to signal safety, respect, and acceptance. As our words diminish in significance and people with dementia become exquisitely attuned to our nonverbal communication, dementia care challenges us to pay attention to what we are communicating. Are our physical demeanor and our words telling the same story? Are stressful factors in our outside lives permeating our interactions with our client? Are we present with the person, actually listening to his or her words and observing his or her behavior, or are our minds somewhere else?

In this fast-paced technological world, health care providers are excellent problem solvers. However, if we get too caught up in interpreting lab and neuropsychological test results we miss the human connection underlying what we are doing. As Monty Roberts (1996) said, "Act like you've only got 15 minutes, it'll take all day [to establish trust]. Act like you've got all day, and it'll only take 15 minutes" (p. 255). Dementia care gives us the opportunity for more mindful and less hurried interactions, and the relationships we build with people with dementia testify to our ability to be present. Learning how to build a genuine human connection with the whole person, rather than by means of cognition alone, can be one of dementia care's greatest rewards.

PERFECTION IS NOT THE GOAL

The second thing that has helped sustain our work over the years is the realization that there is no single "right" way to provide dementia care. The situations and experiences of living with dementia are as varied as snowflakes. The possible contingency relationships—activators and consequences surrounding a behavior of interest—that may be influencing a situation are many and diverse and not always obvious to the outside observer. We sometimes tell caregivers that they are like scientists observing the lions of the Serengeti: Why does the mother lion go to this watering hole and not the other? Why does the care recipient want to stay up all night on Tuesday and hit the sack at 8 p.m. on Saturday? What factors might be influencing these behavior patterns that we just have not figured out? Most likely, there are many contingencies in play with every situation that we are trying to figure out, and there is no one solution to discover. We have to remind caregivers (and ourselves) that not all A • B • C interventions we come up with will work. Sometimes interventions work only intermittently or stop working altogether after a while. The clinician's solution to a problem may be completely ineffective, whereas an idea a caregiver comes up with—which at first seems ridiculous— may work perfectly well. There is no single perfect behavioral intervention, and although we health care professionals may be experts in our subject matter, we are certainly no more expert in figuring out how to help the care recipient in our office than is the caregiver who sits beside him or her.

This is important to remember because we, like the caregivers and care recipients we serve, often feel compelled to have all the answers and to make everything come out all right as quickly as possible. Dementia care, however, is not like giving the proper antibiotic to a patient with pneumonia. It is OK to experiment with interventions and to fail; there is even freedom in both you and the caregiver knowing you do not have to have all the answers. In fact, sometimes the solution to an objective problem is less important than how you make the person with dementia feel. By following the DANCE principles— discussing concerns respectfully, ameliorating excess disability, nurturing the dyad, creating contextual solutions, and enjoying sharing the journey—you can approach each unique situation, each follow-up visit, with a fresh eye and new curiosity about what it can teach you. Generating hypotheses and implementing interventions, we are never "done" or bored; in the words of Dorothy Parker, "The cure for boredom is curiosity. There is no cure for curiosity" (Lewis, 2009). There is always more to spark your curiosity and to learn from persons with dementia; accepting that gift from them will further enrich both you and them.

BUILDING A GOOD SUPPORT SYSTEM

The last thing to remember is that you do not have to go it alone. You need to build on the strength of your colleagues and lean on the support of your friends.

Working with persons with dementia is by its very nature a collaborative venture. The complexity of dementia care leads us to cross paths with colleagues from many disciplines, and all of them—medicine, nursing, social work, physical and occupational therapy, psychology, and pastoral counseling—have something to contribute to enhancing the quality of life for those with a progressive brain disease. Each field has its own scientific explanatory models and valuable perspectives to share. New and more effective intervention and assessment strategies are continually emerging. There is always more to learn about the genetics, neurophysiology, and sociological context of dementia. We have every reason to hope that on the horizon are new and better ways to prevent the onset of behavioral symptoms of dementia, slow their progression, and relieve the suffering they bring. The DANCE principles and model of contextual care that we have introduced in this volume will serve you well as new and improved specialized treatments emerge, helping you work collaboratively with your clients to test treatment efficacy and appropriateness for each unique situation and to reach out to your colleagues to share what you have learned. It has been said that "it takes a village to raise a child," and this statement is equally true at the opposite end of the age spectrum.

Working with persons with dementia also offers an opportunity to grow outside your own personal comfort zone. Behavioral health care in dementia demands constant weighing of worldviews and values such as autonomy versus beneficence and risk versus safety. Coming to know how your assumptions about competence, aging, and conformity influence your responses; overcoming the seemingly reflexive impetus of providing immediate solutions; and establishing collaborations with your clients for creative problem solving are all steps toward personal growth that generalize beyond your daily practice.

However, being outside one's comfort zone can leave you reeling with fatigue, uncertainty, and self-doubt. If you are feeling on the edge, struggling with how to make a difference in your practice, consult with a colleague. Talk to a neutral but experienced and wise caregiver. Surround yourself with friends and loved ones. Laugh with your children. Walk at sunrise with your spouse or partner. Listening to these multiple voices is essential to good dementia care. Dementia health care providers, like family caregivers, need to refuel the emotional batteries from time to time.

CHANGING THE FACE OF DEMENTIA CARE

A German author said, "How a society treats its members with dementia is the crucial test of its humanity" (Lütz, 2009). We have seen throughout this book that working with older adults with dementia is both a challenge and a gift. The challenge is that compared with other professional domains, dementia care is not deemed glamorous or prestigious work. Many of the people we serve are among the forgotten ones of our modern society: the old and frail, the dying, people who have lost their youth, who can no longer toilet themselves, or be counted on to say the right thing in social settings. They may not always appreciate your clinical advice, they may become restless in your waiting room if you are running behind schedule, and they may forget to pay you. You may at times feel helpless, impatient, or discouraged. Yet, you have an opportunity to bring creativity and generosity to situations that initially seem overwhelmingly difficult but are replete with long-term rewards. One of our tasks as behavioral health care providers is to share with others the possibilities in dementia care and to thereby change the perception of the disease and its associated stigma (e.g., "They are only getting worse anyway"). Just as the range of what is considered possible has changed in the care of individuals with developmental disabilities, so it is our goal to change the face of dementia care.

The gift for us, the health care providers, lies in all that these individuals have to teach us, in the experience of collaboration and intimacy, and in the opportunity for personal growth. Older adults' lives are not just "one thing"; no two stories are the same, and no two people experience or cope with difficulties remembering, thinking, or problem solving in the same way. Finding out how dementia affects one particular client, and what dementia means for him or her, invites curiosity, caring, and flexibility on the part of the health care provider. We wrote this book to enable you to tackle the challenge of dementia care and to share with you the many gifts of learning that we have received from our cognitively impaired clients.

Engaging in a contextual model of dementia care is a skill like riding a bicycle: If you are willing to try something new and get on the bicycle, you will little-by-little move along more smoothly. The assessment, referral, and treatment tools we have described in this book are designed to generate flexibility in your responding by providing you with a new care goal. Your job is not to take away the dementia and its related changes. Rather, within the very real situation of cognitive loss and its consequences, you have the opportunity to discover new ways in which individuals with dementia can engage, connect, and enjoy activities as well as others' company. We hope that this book has helped bring you a little closer to that goal.

APPENDIX A: USEFUL ASSESSMENT MEASURES FOR DEMENTIA CARE

These tables are not intended to be an exhaustive listing of instruments or assessment domains important in the evaluation and treatment of cognitively impaired older adults and their caregivers. In particular, a vast number of neuropsychological assessment instruments are in wide use for diagnosing dementia and its subtypes, and a full description of these is beyond the scope of the current book.

TABLE A.1
Common Cognitive, Mood, and Behavioral Screening Instruments Used With Persons With Cognitive Impairment or Dementia

Domain	Measure name	Citation
Agitation	Agitated Behavior in Dementia Scale (ABID)	Logsdon, 1999
	Cohen-Mansfield Agitation Inventory (CMAI)	Cohen-Mansfield, Marx, & Rosenthal, 1989
Anxiety	Rating Anxiety in Dementia (RAID)	Shankar, Walker, Frost, & Orrell, 1999
Cognitive function	Alzheimer's Disease Assessment Center–Cognitive subscale (ADAS-Cog)	Rosen, Mohs, & Davis, 1984
	Clock Drawing Test (CLOX)	Royall, Cordes, & Polk, 1998
	Cognitive Abilities Screening Instrument	Teng et al., 1994
	Dementia Rating Scale 2	Jurica, Leitten, & Mattis, 2002
	Executive Interview (EXIT25)	Royall, Mahurin, & Gray, 1992
	Mini-Cog	Borson, Scanlan, Brush, Vitaliano, & Dokmak, 2000
	Mini-Mental State Examination (MMSE)	Folstein, Folstein, & McHugh, 1975
	Modified Mini-Mental State (3MS)	Teng & Chui, 1987
Depression	Cornell Scale for Depression in Dementia (CSDD)	Alexopoulos, Abrams, Young, & Shamoian, 1988
	Dementia Mood Assessment Scale (DMAS)	Sunderland, Hill, Lawlor, & Molchan, 1988
	Geriatric Depression Scale (GDS)	Yesavage et al., 1983
	Hamilton Depression Rating Scale (DHRS)	Hamilton, 1960
Functional status	Alzheimer's Disease Assessment Center-Functional Assessment Scale (ADAS-FAS)	Thal, 1997
	Direct Assessment of Functional Status (DAFS)	Loewenstein et al., 1989
	Clinical Dementia Rating Scale (CDRS)	Hughes, Berg, Danziger, Coben, & Martin, 1982
	Instrumental Activities of Daily Living Scales (IADL)	Lawton & Brody, 1969
	Physical Self-Maintenance Scale (PSM)	Lawton & Brody, 1969
General behavioral disturbance	Behavioral Pathology in Alzheimer's Disease (BEHAV-AD)	Reisberg et al., 1987
	CERAD Behavior Rating Scale for Dementia (BRSD)	Tariot et al., 1995
	Neuropsychiatric Inventory (NPI)	Cummings et al., 1994
	Revised Memory and Behavior Problem Checklist (RMBPC)	Teri et al., 1992
Sleep	Epworth Sleepiness Scale (ESS)	Johns, 1991
	Sleep Disorders Inventory (SDI)	Tractenberg, Singer, Cummings, & Thal, 2003
	Timed Behavioral Disturbance Questionnaire (TBDQ)	Bliwise, Yesavage, & Tinklenberg, 1992
Quality of life	Quality of Life in Alzheimer's Disease (QOL-AD)	Logsdon, Gibbons, McCurry, & Teri, 1999
	Pleasant Event Schedule-Alzheimer's Disease (PES-AD)	Teri & Logsdon, 1991

TABLE A.2
Common Mood and Behavioral Screening Instruments Used for Caregivers of Persons With Cognitive Impairment or Dementia

Domain	Measure name	Citation
Anxiety	Beck Anxiety Inventory (BAI)	A. T. Beck, Epstein, Brown, & Steer, 1988
	Hamilton Anxiety Rating Scale (HARS)	Hamilton, 1959
Attachment	Measure of Attachment Qualities (MAQ)	Carver, 1997a
Burden	Caregiver Burden Inventory (CBI)	Zarit, Todd, & Zarit, 1986
	Caregiver Strain Index (CSI)	Robinson, 1983
	Perceived Stress Scale (PSS)	Cohen, Kamarck, & Mermelstein, 1983
	Screen for Caregiver Burden (SCB)	Vitaliano, Russo, Young, Becker, & Maiuro, 1991
Competence	Short Sense of Competence Questionnaire (SSCQ)	Vernooij-Dassen et al., 1999
Coping	Brief Coping Orientation to Problems Experienced (Brief COPE)	Carver, 1997b
	Dementia Management Strategies Scale (DMSS)	Hinrichsen & Niederehe, 1995
	Revised Scale for Caregiving Self-Efficacy (RSCSE)	Steffen, McKibbin, Zeiss, Gallagher-Thompson, & Bandura, 2002
Depression	Beck Depression Inventory-II (BDI-II)	A. T. Beck, Steer, & Brown, 1995
	Center for Epidemiological Studies-Depression (CES-D)	Radloff, 1977
	Geriatric Depression Scale (GDS)	Yesavage et al., 1983
	Hamilton Depression Rating Scale (DHRS)	Hamilton, 1960
Quality of life	Life Experiences Survey (LES)	Russo & Vitaliano, 1995
	Medical Outcome Short Form (SF-36) Health Survey	Ware, Snow, Kosinski, & Gandek, 1993
	Pleasant Event Schedule (PES)	Lewinsohn, Muñoz, Youngren, & Zeiss, 1992
	Quality of Life in Alzheimer's Disease (QOL-AD)	Logsdon, Gibbons, et al., 1999
Relationships	Boundary Ambiguity Scale	Boss, Caron, Horbal, & Mortimer, 1990
	Family Assessment Measure (FAM)	Skinner, Steinhauer, & Santa-Barbara, 1983
	Positive Aspects of Caregiving	Schulz et al., 1997
	Miller Social Intimacy Scale (MSIS)	Miller & Lefcourt, 1982
Resilience	Resilience Scale	Wagnild & Young, 1993
General	Caregiver Activities Time Survey (CATS)	Clipp & Moore, 1995
	Expressed Emotion (EE)	Vitaliano, Young, Russo, Romano, & Magana-Amato, 1993
	Positive and Negative Affect Scale (PANAS)	Watson, Clark, & Tellegen, 1988
	Psychiatric Symptom Checklist (SCL-90-R)	Derogatis, 1994

APPENDIX B:
A • B • C TRACKING SHEET

Caregiver name		Target behavior:			Date:
	Activators	Specify the behavior	Consider the consequences		
Date and time of day	*Where and around whom did the behavior occur?*	*What exactly is the person doing that you would like to see change?*	*Immediate: What did the behavior accomplish? How did you respond? What did you think, say, feel, or do?*		
	Consider the broader psychosocial context.	*Gather a history of that specific behavior.*	*General: Conduct a reinforcer assessment.*	*Long-term: Over time, did the behavior increase or decrease?*	

APPENDIX C: SAMPLE CONSULTATION REPORT ILLUSTRATING A CASE CONCEPTUALIZATION

Mrs. Margo Caldwell, Mr. Jeremy Caldwell, and Mrs. Amelia Margate attended two assessment sessions on September 12, 2008.[1] The first session was held at the behavioral health care providers' offices with Mr. and Mrs. Caldwell; the next session took place in the care recipient's home with Mrs. Margate alone. A phone interview was conducted with Ms. Rimini, Elder Protective Services social worker, also on September 12, 2008.

PRESENTING COMPLAINT

Mr. Caldwell is the 47-year-old primary caregiver and the attorney-in-fact of his 66-year-old retired mother, Mrs. Amelia Margate, who was diagnosed with probable dementia of the Alzheimer's type (per reports dated August 5, 2008, by Dr. Neurologist and August 10, 2008, by Dr. Neuropsychologist). According to the primary caregiver, Mrs. Margate still lives independently, without insight into her cognitive deficits. Mr. and Mrs. Caldwell were referred for dementia-related behavioral health services by Ms. Rimini, Elder Protective Services social worker. Mr. and Mrs. Caldwell complained about ongoing conflict with Ms. Margate, related to Ms. Margate's initiation of formal complaint proceedings, repeated utilization of police emergency and Elder Protective Services, her wish and preparation to relocate in Florida, her fearful behavior, and her paranoid beliefs about Mr. and Mrs. Caldwell.

DETAILED PRESENTING COMPLAINTS, PER PRIMARY CAREGIVER INTERVIEW

Repeated Complaint Proceedings and Use of Emergency Services

The primary caregiver reported that approximately 1 year ago, Ms. Margate's power was shut off because of her failure to pay her bills. She began to believe that the U.S. Postal Service delivered her mail to her neighbors and initiated a series of complaints via phone calls, letters, and e-mails to state

---

[1]This is a fully de-identified report; like the other case examples in this book, all names, dates, and potentially identifying details are fictitious.

and federal agencies. Subsequent difficulties balancing her bank accounts resulted in a similar string of formal complaints, this time directed at banking officials and reaching the state government level. As Ms. Margate's organizational and planning deficits increased, household items, financial tools such as credit cards or checkbooks, and other important items (car registration, proof of insurance, health insurance) went missing and reappeared, seemingly unpredictably. Ms. Margate found herself in constant conflict with utility and other providers (cable, phone, health insurance), who were threatening to terminate services. Within the last 3 months, Ms. Margate has made approximately fifty 911 calls regarding break-ins and theft. She also has contacted state and federal agencies as well as Elder Protective Services to complain about what she calls the local police's inertia and lackadaisical attitude toward their duty to protect senior citizens.

Preparation to Relocate to Florida

Ms. Margate used to live at 2769 Heath Street in Jacksonville, Florida. According to her son, Ms. Margate is convinced she would gain police protection and peace of mind by moving to 2769 Heath Street. She has ordered moving boxes, started packing the household, and has called AAA to service her car for the long trip home (although Mr. Caldwell had disconnected the car battery to prevent her departure). She has also entered into contracts with three different realtors to sell her current home and is in touch with a Jacksonville realtor to repurchase her old home.

Fearful and Self-Protective Behavior

The primary caregiver reported that he removed a handgun with which Ms. Margate had slept at night. He said Ms. Margate was barricading the doors to her bedroom with furniture and sleeps with an axe and a hammer in her bed and a pitchfork nearby. Ms. Margate showed those items to the coaches during the home visit and maintained she saw a man standing at the foot of her bed and watching her at night. Ms. Margate had the locks to her house changed more than a dozen times within the last 2 months.

Accusatory and Threatening Behavior

Ms. Margate has accused her family caregivers of financial exploitation. Since Mr. Caldwell took her to a neurologist and a neuropsychologist, Ms. Margate has forbidden her son access to her house, saying that her son bribed an "impostor" to act as a physician, declare her incompetent, and have her committed. During the home visit, she threatened her son and the professionals with litigation and physical violence ("punching his lights out"). She also reported that the "man at the foot of her bed" refrained from attacking her because she screamed loudly and jumped toward him to land a punch.

PSYCHOSOCIAL AND RELATIONSHIP HISTORY

According to the primary caregiver's report, Ms. Margate grew up in Florida, where her father's family had considerable wealth. Ms. Margate experienced childhood physical abuse by her father. She graduated from high school. Pregnant at 18, she married Mr. Caldwell's father, whom she divorced 5 years later. Upon the divorce, she reassumed her birth name, entered college, became a teacher, and raised Mr. Caldwell alone. Mr. Caldwell described his relationship with his mother as "very close." Ms. Margate inherited her parents' estate when Mr. Caldwell was about 10 years old. He recalled travels abroad, studies, and many leisure activities (e.g., art exhibition, museum, concert visits) with his mother. Ms. Margate retired from teaching 12 years ago. According to Mr. Caldwell, she "made too many errors." A year later, Ms. Margate moved from Florida to join Mr. Caldwell and his family out of state. For the past 6 months, Mr. Caldwell and Ms. Margate have argued about her plans to return to Florida. Since Mr. Caldwell has taken Ms. Margate for cognitive evaluations, she has not permitted him access to her home.

QUALITY OF CURRENT CAREGIVER–CARE RECIPIENT RELATIONSHIP

During the home visit, Ms. Margate immediately started talking about her son and how much his seemingly "treacherous" behavior had disappointed her. She cried when mentioning Mr. Caldwell's name. Mr. Caldwell said that his wife, who visited Ms. Margate once a day to perform household chores and drop off groceries, had a better relationship with Ms. Margate than he currently did. During the home visit, Ms. Margate said she did her own shopping and did not mention her daughter-in-law.

FAMILY HISTORY OF DEMENTIA

Ms. Margate's mother had dementia, possibly of the Alzheimer's type. Ms. Margate placed her in a nursing home. Ms. Margate's mother passed away in her late 50s.

CHART REVIEW OF CARE RECIPIENT
PSYCHIATRIC AND MEDICAL HISTORY

Aside from recent information obtained by Dr. Neurologist and Dr. Neuropsychologist, no records are available for review. Mr. Caldwell reported that Ms. Margate had requested her records from her physicians in Florida when she relocated. The physicians heeded Ms. Margate's request, but the records have since been lost. According to Mr. Caldwell, Ms. Margate was diagnosed with chronic depression 11 years ago and retired from teaching with disability due to chronic depression. She received a diagnosis of dementia consistent with the Alzheimer's type from Dr. Neurologist on August 5, 2008 (MMSE = 17), and from Dr. Neuropsychologist on August 10, 2008 (see next section). In terms of other medically relevant events, Ms. Margate had a traumatic brain injury in early childhood (at 7 years old, according to Mr. Caldwell's report). Mr. Caldwell reported Ms. Margate had been "comatose." According to Mr. Caldwell, Ms. Margate does not have any allergies; her vision is corrected (glasses for myopia), and her hearing is intact; her coordination is intact, and her gait is of normal velocity and narrow based.

CHART REVIEW OF CARE RECIPIENT
COGNITIVE ABILITY

Dr. Neuropsychologist's report of August 10, 2008, suggests that Mrs. Margate's strengths are reading, language ability, and verbal attention. Attention was impaired when basic attentional capacity was assessed by predominantly nonverbal means (e.g., distraction counting). Mental status tests and the Dementia Rating Scale-2 revealed significant deficits in episodic memory, visuospatial, and executive functioning, with relative preservation of language and memory of distant past events. These findings are consistent with the clinical impression based upon behavioral observations and Dr. Neurologist's report.

CHART REVIEW OF CARE RECIPIENT
MEDICATION STATUS

No records are available for review. Mr. Caldwell reported that his mother had a history of taking antiseizure medication related to the traumatic brain injury. He said that she stopped taking the medication approximately 3 years ago and had refused any prescription medication since.

CARE RECIPIENT SLEEP, CONTINENCE, AND NUTRITIONAL STATUS

Ms. Margate and Mr. Caldwell report that Ms. Margate's sleep is disrupted. She is continent. Her weight has decreased by more than 15 lb within the last 6 months, prompting nutritional concerns.

CARE RECIPIENT AFFECT, BEHAVIOR, AND COGNITION

Mental Status

Ms. Margate was alert but not fully oriented to time, location, role, or purpose during the home visit.

Mood and Behavior

Ms. Margate was very tearful at times, repeatedly expressing her belief that her son was making plans to institutionalize her or to legally forfeit her personhood. Tears alternated with laughter and hopefulness about living at 2769 Heath Street in Florida, reconnecting with old neighbors, and finding safety in a familiar neighborhood "where the police care."

At one time during the home visit, Ms. Margate said she urgently needed her "contact lens solution" and began a frantic, fast-past search throughout the house. The coaches noticed that Ms. Margate was wearing her glasses and not her contacts. Being told to touch her face and feel her glasses, Ms. Margate angrily said to the coaches, "I think you do not understand. My contacts are drying on my eyes as we speak. I may have to take a gun and shoot you." The coaches apologized for their misinterpretation of the situation and then assisted her in searching for the "contact lens solution," which turned out to be a small 50-ml bottle of saline solution for dry eyes. Ms. Margate seemed relieved, appropriately thanked the coaches for their help, and returned to friendly conversation without seeming recollection of the event or her threat.

When not talking about perceived break-ins and exploitation, Ms. Margate's affect was jovial and very pleasant. She engaged in lively conversation despite her inability to remember recent events. She smiled frequently, had a sense of humor, and recited to the visiting behavioral health coaches facts about geography and history.

Cognition

Her memory was severely impaired. Although she was able to repeat 4/4 words, after 5 min she guessed none of them from multiple choice or prompting. She was unable to draw a floor plan of her house and gave up after drawing two lines. When asked to draw a clock, she drew a very small dot (without numbers on the inside or outside of the circle) and was unable to draw the hands. She was able to mimic simple hand symbols (victory sign, A-OK sign) but unable to mimic more complex ones. Language seemed within normal limits; she could name, repeat, write, and read. Her speech was fluent though vague and tangential. Her range of conversational topics was limited to her son's behavior, returning to Florida, and the perceived break-ins.

Behavioral Strengths

When Ms. Margate felt safe and was not overwhelmed by her memory deficits, she showed caring, empathy, and social skills. She frequently talked about herself as a person who "will stand up for herself," yet will forgive others (e.g., students) as long as they confess to their omissions or wrongdoings, such as forgetting homework or cheating on tests. She was sensitive to any social degradation. Her history of being a teacher and having access to significant financial resources seemed to contribute to Ms. Margate's willingness to take charge and solve problems. Ms. Margate cares about her appearance (e.g., commenting that she has techniques for keeping her long hair shiny, stating she knows she looks young, wearing nail polish).

Pleasant Events

Ms. Margate enjoys (a) being given choices; (b) problem solving; (c) conversations, including those about experiences traveling abroad, geography, history, and Florida; (d) walking; (e) gardening; (f) dining; (g) professional care (hair, manicures, pedicures).

HOME CONDITION

Ms. Margate lives in a single-story ranch house, which is appropriate considering her severe visuospatial deficits; there are no stairs in the house or leading to it. The floor is carpeted in a uniform color throughout the house. The household is partially packed in boxes that are stacked in an open living room/dining area. There is no evidence of food preparation in the kitchen. Ms. Margate's bedroom suite contains household items from all over the house, stacked and piled in a manner that a virtual obstacle course is created. Ms. Margate's bed seems to serve as shelving or receptacle for household items and tools with which Ms. Margate says she sleeps, including an axe, a hammer in the bed, and a pitchfork next to it. There are potentially disorienting large mirrors in the bedroom. Ms. Margate's bathroom is connected to her bedroom and might not be easily located by her, given the cluttered environment. Safety devices, such as handrails in the shower or within reach of the toilet, are missing. Ms. Margate reported she spent most of her day in her office, the floor of which is covered with files and papers. Bundles of unopened mail are on shelves, and the desk area, including the computer monitor and its surroundings, is covered with Post-it notes. Business cards, including one from Elder Protective Services and two from police detectives, are taped to the bureau.

CAREGIVER MEDICAL STATUS

The primary caregiver describes his health as "good" and reports Type 2 diabetes and hypertension. According to him, his conditions are managed with drugs (metformin, amlodipin, respectively).

CAREGIVER MOOD, AFFECT, AND BEHAVIOR

Mr. Caldwell expressed both embarrassment and concern over his mother's behavior. He said he was initially angry about his mother's "stubborn" and "obstinate" adherence to her plan to relocate in Florida, about the complaints, the calls to emergency responders, and the accusations.

Instrumental Caregiving Tasks and Skills

Caregiving Tasks

Mr. Caldwell has rerouted Ms. Margate's mail to his address and is now managing her finances with quarterly oversight from social services. As recently as September of 2008, he transported Ms. Margate to doctors' appointments and to church. Mrs. Caldwell drops off groceries at Ms. Margate's house and performs daily wellness checks.

Caregiving Skills

The primary caregiver tends to rely on reasoning and persuasion to affect Ms. Margate's behavior. Like many caregivers, he has difficulty understanding the care recipient's inability to understand instructions and lack of reasoning, organizing, and planning ability when language is largely preserved. Thus, Ms. Margate's relatively spared language abilities contribute to the caregivers' difficulties in engaging with Ms. Margate in a dementia-appropriate manner. Both caregivers tend to describe Ms. Margate's behavior as "intentional" and "part of her personality" rather than attributing it to Ms. Margate's profound deficits in problem solving and remembering. The primary caregiver in particular does not seem to view Ms. Margate's behavior as a reaction to frightening situations (e.g., inability to find familiar objects, visual disturbances) or social interactions that she interprets as demeaning, coercive, or belittling. The primary caregiver also seems unaware that his physical demeanor (i.e., increased frustration when instructions are not followed, anger about Ms. Margate's insistence to return to 2769 Heath Street, as indicated by tone of voice, facial expression, and posture) may function to generate further fearful and self-protective behaviors. According to the caregivers' report, Ms. Margate will not permit him access to her home. Hired professional caregivers may be more skillful in their approach toward Ms. Margate. Moreover, they do not have a history of aversive interactions with Ms. Margate that lead to perceived negative outcomes for her (e.g., admission to a facility).

The primary caregiver is a generally competent individual and, as a result, may not ask for help needed to learn to effectively communicate with Ms. Margate. He has to date tended toward emotional responding when efforts to intervene are unsuccessful, rather than goal-directed problem solving.

COMMUNITY AND SOCIAL SUPPORT RESOURCES AND NEEDS

Ms. Margate reported that she missed attending church services. Ms. Margate's deficits have isolated her socially, and she would benefit from reintegration into a dementia-appropriate social environment.

HYPOTHETICAL FUNCTION OF BEHAVIORS

Repeated Complaint Proceedings and Use of Emergency Services

Ms. Margate's lack of insight into her deficits may render her difficulties managing her affairs of daily living virtually insurmountable. Both the complaint proceedings and the use of emergency services may function to rationalize and make sense out of financial mismanagement and other problems. In addition, Ms. Margate is socially isolated. Telephone contacts with agencies may be her only current social resource.

Preparation to Relocate in Florida

Ms. Margate's wish to return to Florida seems to reflect a wish to have things "as they used to be," namely, predictable, safe, and simple. The wish to return to Florida may be a description of how overwhelming Ms. Margate's current living situation is.

Fearful and Self-Protective Behaviors

Ms. Margate's visual disturbances, combined with her memory loss and lack of organizational skills, may prompt her self-protective behavior, particularly at night.

Accusatory Behaviors Toward Mr. Caldwell

Ms. Margate's accusations may function (a) to engage others in conversations and hold their attention, given Ms. Margate's limited range of communicative topics; (b) to help Ms. Margate make sense of the neurological and neuropsychological assessments, given her lack of insight; (c) to help Ms. Margate make sense of actual, recent events, such as the lack of mail which has been rerouted to her son's house; and (d) to help Ms. Margate make sense of the caregivers' worried, angry, or frustrated physical demeanor and facial expressions even when they are unrelated to her, given her limited ability to understand the purpose of other people's behavior.

Threatening Verbal Behaviors

Ms. Margate's inability to reason may result in threats (e.g., toward the coaches in the context of finding eye drops, toward the physicians and her sons). She may escape other people's attempts to orient her to reality by verbally "bullying" them to stop. Given Ms. Margate's inability to consider more than one alternative at the same time, the threats may thus have a self-protective and purely verbal–communicative function.

CARE PLAN

Given Ms. Margate's considerable deficits, independent living seems distressing and overwhelming. It may also contribute to Ms. Margate's fearfulness and her self-protective behavior, as well as her accusatory and threatening behavior. Ms. Margate is pleasant and cooperative as long as she is approached in a respectful and dignified manner. She may react with formal complaints, emergency calls, fear and self-protective behaviors, accusations and threats if (a) she encounters consequences of her cognitive deficits (e.g., unpaid bills), (b) she is oriented to reality, (c) she is not given choices, (d) she is offered assistance in a way that points to her deficits, (e) persuasion is used and she cannot follow the reasoning; (f) she "reads" angry or frustrated facial expressions; and (g) coercive means are used to achieve compliance. In general, Ms. Margate will collaborate with requests for help and accept apologies.

Relocation

Ms. Margate may benefit from relocation to a dementia-appropriate environment as soon as possible. The coaches will assist the caregiver in selecting an appropriate facility and work with the family and the professional caregivers to facilitate Ms. Margate's relocation. The coaches will take Ms. Margate to the facility for a family-style meal, observe her behavior within that context, and aid her remaining at the facility using compassionate misinformation. The misinformation will be derived from Ms. Margate's interpretation of the dementia-appropriate environment (e.g., college dorm, hotel, association, condominium as a gift, apartment in Florida). It is not expected that Ms. Margate will be aware of the purpose, role, or location of a dementia-appropriate facility.

Dementia Education

The caregiver and his wife may benefit from dementia education, including communication training and behavioral management with individuals with dementia. To facilitate the interaction with Ms. Margate, to effectively advocate for her, and to transition her to a specialized dementia care unit, the family caregivers must learn to understand her behavior as a joint function of her history, the current social context, and her cognitive deficits. A detailed review of Ms. Margate's test performances will be scheduled with the caregivers to contextualize Ms. Margate's behaviors. Family caregivers must obtain the skills to deescalate Ms. Margate to keep her safe (e.g., apologizing for the situation, taking the blame, allowing Ms. Margate to maintain her beliefs about the situation).

Emotional Support

Reestablishing the close relationship between Ms. Margate and her son will be the focus of emotional support. The coaches will also provide support to Mr. Caldwell, Ms. Margate, and professional staff during the transition.

Instrumental Support

The family and professional caregivers may benefit from the following strategies.

Modeling

The coaches will model how to interact with Ms. Margate without occasioning self-protective behavior. They will emphasize Ms. Margate's lack of insight into her deficits and stress others' apologies, taking the blame, and providing Ms. Margate with a dignified escape from difficult situations.

Shaping and Instructing

The coaches will reinforce appropriate care and advocacy by the caregivers and instruct performance, if necessary.

Discrimination Training

The coaches will point out situations to the family and professional caregivers in which to advocate for Ms. Margate and in which to ask for assistance.

In-the-Moment Coaching

The caregivers will be encouraged to use the 24/7 helpline to receive instrumental support in situations of developing conflict with Ms. Margate.

Socialization

Ms. Margate will be enrolled in the companion program, with the goal to arrange supervised walks and facilitate transition to a locked environment.

As with all individuals with dementia, Ms. Margate will thrive in any environment she perceives as safe (i.e., in which she is treated with respect and affection, is given limited and safe access to choices, and in which she does not have to confront her deficits). Given Ms. Margate's difficulties in her home environment, we recommend that placement in a specialized dementia care unit will be effected as soon as possible.

September 24, 2008

APPENDIX D:
ADDITIONAL RESOURCES

- *Administration on Aging.* U.S. Department of Health and Human Services site providing information about home and community-based services that help elderly individuals maintain their health and independence in their homes and communities. Website: http://www.aoa.gov
- *Area Agencies on Aging* (AAA). Offices in every state provide information and assistance regarding local resources for older adults, including Aging and Adult Services, Senior Information and Assistance, and Adult Protective Services. These agencies can also assist in applying for Medicaid. Website: http://www.n4a.org/
- *Alzheimer's Association.* Offers information about support groups, educational programs and materials, case management, and community resources for AD patients and caregivers. Website: http://www.alz.org
- *Alzheimer's Disease Education and Referral Center* (ADEAR). Provides educational materials and information produced by the National Institute on Aging and Alzheimer's Disease Research Centers. Website: http://www.nia.nih.gov/alzheimers
- *American Association for Retired Persons* (AARP). Provides general information on topics pertinent to persons over age 55, including a link to family caregiving topics. Website: http://www.aarp.org
- *American Health Assistance Foundation* (AHAF). Includes information about Alzheimer's disease family relief program. Website: http://www.ahaf.org
- *ElderCare Online.* On-line informational booklets, resources, support groups, and products for all aspects of Alzheimer's and dementia care. Website: http://www.ec-online.net/alzchannel.htm
- *Mayo Clinic Health Page.* Nationally recognized Web page with links to health topics including Alzheimer's disease and an "ask the expert" page. Website: http://www.mayoclinic.com
- *Medicare.* Ask Medicare caregiver site provides information about the spectrum of caregiver support resources available for caregivers. Website: http://www.medicare.gov/caregivers/

- *National Alliance for Caregiving* (NAC). A nonprofit coalition of national organizations focused on caregiving issues. Website: http://www.caregiving.org
- *National Association of Professional Geriatric Care Managers.* Geriatric care managers may be nurses, social workers, or other professionals trained in assessing an individual's needs and making appropriate recommendations. This is an especially good resource for families that do not live in the same town as the patient or for caregivers that are overwhelmed. Website: http://www.caremanager.org
- *National Clearinghouse for Long-Term Care Information.* Site sponsored by the U.S. Department of Health and Human Services to provide information and resources to help you and your family plan for future long-term care needs. Website: http://www.longtermcare.gov/LTC/Main_Site/index.aspx
- *National Family Caregivers Association.* A caregiver advocacy site to provide education and support to Americans caring for loved ones with a chronic illness, disability, or the frailties of old age. Website: http://www.nfcacares.org/
- *National Institutes of Health (NIH) registry of clinical trials.* Compiles federally and privately supported clinical trials being conducted around with world, with information about the purpose, location, and recruitment of ongoing clinical trials, as well as about consumer health. Website: http://www.ClinicalTrials.gov
- *NIHSeniorHealth.* Provides information through the NIH on a wide range of health related topics, with links to Alzheimer's disease and caregiving. Website: http://www.nihseniorhealth.gov
- *Psychologists in Long-term Care, Inc.* Professional networking, information, and advocacy. Website: http://www.pltcweb.org
- *U.S. National Library of Medicine.* Provides health news and link lists of health libraries, databases, and resources. Websites: http://www.ncbi.nlm.nih.gov/pubmed/ and http://www.medlineplus.gov

REFERENCES

Albert, S. M., Del Castillo-Castaneda, C., Sano, M., Jacobs, D. M., Marder, K., Bell, K., . . . Stern, Y. (1996). Quality of life in patients with Alzheimer's disease as reported by patient proxies. *Journal of the American Geriatrics Society, 44*, 1342–1347.

Alexopoulos, G. S., Abrams, R. C., Young, R. C., & Shamoian, C. A. (1988). Cornell Scale for Depression in Dementia. *Biological Psychiatry, 23*, 271–284. doi:10.1016/0006-3223(88)90038-8

Algase, D. L., Beck, C., Kolawnowski, A., Whall, A., Berent, S., Richards, K., . . . Beattie, E. (1996). Need-driven dementia-compromised behavior (NDB): An alternative view of disruptive behavior. *American Journal of Alzheimer's Disease and Other Dementias, 11*(6), 10–19. doi:10.1177/153331759601100603

American Academy of Neurology, Ethics, and Humanities Subcommittee. (1996). Ethical issues in the management of the demented patient. *Neurology, 46*, 1180–1183.

American Psychiatric Association. (2000). *Diagnostic and statistical manual of mental disorders* (4th ed., text rev.). Washington, DC: Author.

American Geriatrics Society and American Association for Geriatric Psychiatry. (2003a). The American Geriatrics Society and American Association for Geriatric Psychiatry recommendations for policies in support of quality mental health care in U.S. nursing homes. *Journal of the American Geriatrics Society, 51*, 1299–1304. doi:10.1046/j.1532-5415.2003.51416.x

American Geriatrics Society and American Association for Geriatric Psychiatry. (2003b). Consensus statement on improving the quality of mental health care in U.S. nursing homes: Management of depression and behavioral symptoms associated with dementia. *Journal of the American Geriatrics Society, 51*, 1287–1298. doi:10.1046/j.1532-5415.2003.51415.x

Aneshensel, C. S., Botticello, A. L., & Yamamoto-Mitani, N. (2004). When caregiving ends: The course of depressive symptoms after bereavement. *Journal of Health and Social Behavior, 45*(4), 422–440. doi:10.1177/002214650404500405

Antipsychotic drugs for dementia: A balancing act. (2009). *Lancet Neurology, 8*(2), 151–157.

Avorn, J., & Wang, P. (2005). Drug prescribing, adverse reactions, and compliance in elderly patients. In C. Salzman (Ed.), *Clinical geriatric psychopharmacology* (4th ed., pp. 23–47). Philadelphia, PA: Lippincott Williams & Wilkins.

Ayalon, L., Gum, A. M., Felician, L., & Arean, P. A. (2006). Effectiveness of nonpharmacological interventions for the management of neuropsychiatric symptoms in patients with dementia. *Archives of Internal Medicine, 166*, 2182–2188. doi:10.1001/archinte.166.20.2182

Ballard, C., Hanney, M. L., Theodoulou, M., Douglas, S., McShane, R., Kossakowski, K., . . . Jacoby, R. (2009). The dementia antipsychotic withdrawal trial (DART-AD): Long-term follow-up of a randomised placebo-controlled trial. *Lancet Neurology, 8*(2), 151–157. doi:10.1016/S1474-4422(08)70295-3

Bechara, A., Tranel, D., Damasio, H., Adolphs, R., Rockland, C., & Damasio, A. R. (1995, August). Double dissociation of conditioning and declarative knowledge relative to the amygdala and hippocampus in humans. *Science, 269,* 1115–1118. doi:10.1126/science.7652558

Beck, A. T., Epstein, N., Brown, G., & Steer, R. A. (1988). An inventory for measuring clinical anxiety: Psychometric properties. *Journal of Consulting and Clinical Psychology, 56,* 893–897. doi:10.1037/0022-006X.56.6.893

Beck, A. T., Steer, R. A., & Brown, G. K. (1995). *Manual for the Beck Depression Inventory–II.* San Antonio, TX: Psychological Corporation.

Beck, C. K., Vogelpohl, T. S., Rasin, J. H., Uriri, J. T., O'Sullivan, P., Walls, R., . . . Baldwin, B. (2002). Effects of behavioral interventions on disruptive behavior and affect in demented nursing home residents. *Nursing Research, 51,* 219–228. doi:10.1097/00006199-200207000-00002

Bell, V., & Troxel, D. (2003). *The best friends approach to Alzheimer's care.* Baltimore, MD: Health Professions Press.

Bick, K. (1999). The early story of Alzheimer disease. In R. D. Terry, R. Katzman, K. L. Bick, & S. S. Sisodia (Eds.), *Alzheimer disease* (2nd ed., pp. 1–9). Philadelphia, PA: Lippincott Williams & Wilkins.

Biglan, A., & Hayes, S. C. (1996). Should the behavioral sciences become more pragmatic? The case for functional contextualism in research on human behavior. *Applied and Preventive Psychology, 5,* 47–57. doi:10.1016/S0962-1849(96)80026-6

Bliwise, D. L., Yesavage, J. A., & Tinklenberg, J. R. (1992). Sundowning and rate of decline in mental function in Alzheimer's disease. *Dementia (Basel, Switzerland), 3,* 335–341.

Bloom, H. G., Ahmed, I., Alessi, C. A., Ancoli-Israel, S., Buysse, D. J., Kryger, M. H., . . . Zee, P. C. (2009). Evidence-based recommendations for the assessment and management of sleep disorders in older persons. *Journal of the American Geriatrics Society, 57,* 761–789. doi:10.1111/j.1532-5415.2009.02220.x

Borson, S., Scanlan, J., Brush, M., Vitaliano, P., & Dokmak, A. (2000). The Mini-Cog: A cognitive "vital signs" measure for dementia screening in multilingual elderly. *International Journal of Geriatric Psychiatry, 15*(11), 1021–1027. doi:10.1002/1099-1166(200011)15:11<1021::AID-GPS234>3.0.CO;2-6

Boss, P., Caron, W., Horbal, J., & Mortimer, J. (1990). Predictors of depression in dementia patients: Boundary ambiguity and mastery. *Family Process, 29*(3), 245–254. doi:10.1111/j.1545-5300.1990.00245.x

Brodaty, H., Green, A., & Koschera, A. (2003). Meta-analysis of psychosocial interventions for caregivers of people with dementia. *Journal of the American Geriatrics Society, 51,* 657–664. doi:10.1034/j.1600-0579.2003.00210.x

Buckley, C., & Estrin, J. (2009, June 14). All-night care for dementia's restless minds. *The New York Times*, p. MB1.

Buckwalter, K. C. (1998). *PLST model: Effectiveness for rural ADRD caregivers. Final report* (R01-NR0234). Washington, DC: National Institute for Nursing Research.

Buckwalter, K. C., Gerdner, L., Kohout, F., Hall, G. R., Kelly, A., Richards, B., ... Sime, M. (1999). A nursing intervention to decrease depression in family caregivers of persons with dementia. *Archives of Psychiatric Nursing, 13*(2), 80–88. doi:10.1016/S0883-9417(99)80024-7

Burgio, L. D., Hardin, J. M., Sinnott, J., Janosky, J., & Hohman, M. J. (1995). Nurses' acceptance of behavioral treatments and pharmacotherapy for behavioral disturbances in older adults. *Applied Nursing Research, 8*(4), 174–181. doi:10.1016/S0897-1897(95)80393-9

Burns, A., Lawlor, B., & Craig, S. (2002). Rating scales in old age psychiatry. *The British Journal of Psychiatry, 180*, 161–167. doi:10.1192/bjp.180.2.161

Burton, L. C., Newsom, J. T., Schulz, R., Hirsch, C. H., & German, P. S. (1997). Preventive health behaviors among spousal caregivers. *Preventive Medicine, 26*, 162–169. doi:10.1006/pmed.1996.0129

Cariaga, J., Burgio, L., Flynn, W., & Martin, D. (1991). A controlled study of disruptive vocalizations among geriatric residents in nursing homes. *Journal of the American Geriatrics Society, 39*, 501–507.

Carver, C. S. (1997a). Adult attachment and personality: Converging evidence and a new measure. *Personality and Social Psychology Bulletin, 23*, 865–883. doi:10.1177/0146167297238007

Carver, C. S. (1997b). You want to measure coping but your protocol's too long: Consider the brief COPE. *International Journal of Behavioral Medicine, 4*, 92–100. doi:10.1207/s15327558ijbm0401_6

Chiesa, M. (1994). *Radical behaviorism: The philosophy and the science*. Boston, MA: Authors Cooperative.

Clipp, E. C., & Moore, M. J. (1995). Caregiver time use: An outcome measure in clinical trial research on Alzheimer's disease. *Clinical Pharmacology and Therapeutics, 58*, 228–236. doi:10.1016/0009-9236(95)90201-5

Cohen-Mansfield, J. (2000). Theoretical frameworks for behavioral problems in dementia. *Alzheimer's Care Quarterly, 1*, 8–21.

Cohen-Mansfield, J., Marx, M. S., & Rosenthal, A. S. (1989). A description of agitation in a nursing home. *Journals of Gerontology, 44*(3), M77–M84.

Cohen, S., Kamarck, T., & Mermelstein, R. (1983). A global measure of perceived stress. *Journal of Health and Social Behavior, 24*(4), 385–396. doi:10.2307/2136404

Cole, C. S., & Richards, K. C. (2006). Sleep in persons with dementia: Increasing quality of life by managing sleep disorders. *Journal of Gerontological Nursing, 32*(3), 48–53.

Cooke, D. D., McNally, L., Mulligan, K. T., Harrison, M. J., & Newman, S. P. (2001). Psychosocial interventions for caregivers of people with dementia:

A systematic review. *Aging & Mental Health, 5*(2), 120–135. doi:10.1080/713650019

Cummings, J. L., Mega, M., Gray, K., Rosenberg-Thompson, S., Carusi, D. A., & Gornbein, J. (1994). The Neuropsychiatric Inventory: Comprehensive assessment of psychopathology in dementia. *Neurology, 44,* 2308–2314.

Davis, R. (1989). *My journey into Alzheimer's disease.* Wheaton, IL: Tyndale House Publishers.

Derogatis, L. R. (1994). *SCL-90-R: Administration, scoring and procedures manual.* Minneapolis, MN: National Computer Systems.

Dettmore, D., Kolanowski, A., & Boustani, M. (2009). Aggression in persons with dementia: Use of nursing theory to guide clinical practice. *Geriatric Nursing, 30,* 8–17. doi:10.1016/j.gerinurse.2008.03.001

Devanand, D. P., Michaels-Marston, K. S., Liu, X., Pelton, G. H., Padilla, M., Marder, K., . . . Mayeux, R. (2000). Olfactory deficits in patients with mild cognitive impairment predict Alzheimer's disease at follow-up. *The American Journal of Psychiatry, 157,* 1399–1405. doi:10.1176/appi.ajp.157.9.1399

de Vugt, M. E., Stevens, F., Aalten, P., Lousberg, R., Jaspers, N., Winkens, I., . . . Verhey, F. R. J. (2003). Behavioural disturbances in dementia patients and quality of the marital relationship. *International Journal of Geriatric Psychiatry, 18*(2), 149–154. doi:10.1002/gps.807

Doody, R. S., Stevens, J. C., Beck, C., Dubinsky, R. M., Kaye, J. A., Gwyther, L., . . . Cummings, J. L. (2001). Practice parameter: Management of dementia (an evidence-based review). Report of the Quality Standards Subcommittee of the American Academy of Neurology. *Neurology, 56,* 1154–1166.

Dowling, J. R. (1995). *Keeping busy: A handbook of activities for persons with dementia.* Baltimore, MD: Johns Hopkins University Press.

Eifert, G. H., & Forsyth, J. P. (2005). *Acceptance and commitment therapy for anxiety disorders.* Oakland, CA: New Harbinger Publications.

Eldridge, L. L., Masterman, D., & Knowlton, B. J. (2002). Intact implicit habit learning in Alzheimer's disease. *Behavioral Neuroscience, 116,* 722–726. doi:10.1037/0735-7044.116.4.722

Emre, M., Aarsland, D., Brown, R., Burn, D. J., Duyckaerts, C., Mizuno, Y., . . . Dubois, B. (2007). Clinical diagnostic criteria for dementia associated with Parkinson's disease. *Movement Disorders, 22,* 1689–1707. doi:10.1002/mds.21507

Esterling, B. A., Kiecolt-Glaser, J. K., Bodnar, J. C., & Glaser, R. (1994). Chronic stress, social support, and persistent alterations in the natural killer cell response to cytokines in older adults. *Health Psychology, 13*(4), 291–298. doi:10.1037/0278-6133.13.4.291

Ferster, C. B. (1973). A functional analysis of depression. *American Psychologist, 28,* 857–870. doi:10.1037/h0035605

Festa, J. R., & Lazar, R. M. (Eds.). (2009). *Neurovascular neuropsychology.* New York, NY: Springer.

Folstein, M. F., Folstein, S. E., & McHugh, P. R. (1975). "Mini-mental state": A practical method for grading the cognitive state of patients for the clinician. *Journal of Psychiatric Research, 12,* 189–198. doi:10.1016/0022-3956(75)90026-6

Friman, P. C., Hayes, S. C., & Wilson, K. G. (1998). Why behavior analysts should study emotion: The example of anxiety. *Journal of Applied Behavior Analysis, 31,* 137–156. doi:10.1901/jaba.1998.31-137

Garand, L., Buckwalter, K. C., Lubaroff, D., Tripp-Reimer, T., Frantz, R. A., & Ansley, T. N. (2002). A pilot study of immune and mood outcomes of a community-based intervention for dementia caregivers: The PLST intervention. *Archives of Psychiatric Nursing, 16*(4), 156–167. doi:10.1053/apnu.2002.34392

Gates, G. A., Anderson, M. L., Feeney, M. P., McCurry, S. M., & Larson, E. B. (2008). Central auditory dysfunction in older persons with memory impairment or Alzheimer dementia. *Archives of Otolaryngology–Head & Neck Surgery, 134,* 771–777. doi:10.1001/archotol.134.7.771

Genova, L. (2009). *Still Alice.* New York, NY: Pocket Books.

Gentry, R. A., & Fisher, J. E. (2007). Conversations in elderly persons with Alzheimer's disease. *Clinical Gerontologist, 31*(2), 77–98. doi:10.1300/J018v31n02_06

Gerdner, L. A., Buckwalter, K. C., & Reed, D. (2002). Impact of a psychoeducational intervention on caregiver response to behavioral problems. *Nursing Research, 51*(6), 363–374. doi:10.1097/00006199-200211000-00004

Gerdner, L. A., Hall, G. R., & Buckwalter, K. C. (1996). Caregiver training for people with Alzheimer's based on a stress threshold model. *The Journal of Nursing Scholarship, 28*(3), 241–246. doi:10.1111/j.1547-5069.1996.tb00358.x

Gifford, E. V., & Hayes, S. C. (1999). Functional contextualism: A pragmatic philosophy for behavioral science. In W. O'Donohue & R. Kitchener (Eds.), *Handbook of behaviorism* (pp. 285–327). San Diego, CA: Academic Press. doi:10.1016/B978-012524190-8/50012-7

Gill, S. S., Mamdani, M., Naglie, G., Streiner, D. L., Bronskill, S. E., Kopp, A., . . . Rochon, P. A. (2005). A prescribing cascade involving cholinesterase inhibitors and anticholinergic drugs. *Archives of Internal Medicine, 165,* 808–813. doi:10.1001/archinte.165.7.808

Gouin, J. P., Hantsoo, L., & Kiecolt-Glaser, J. K. (2008). Immune dysregulation and chronic stress among older adults: A review. *Neuroimmunomodulation, 15*(4–6), 251–259. doi:10.1159/000156468

Graves, A. B., Bowen, J. D., Rajaram, L., McCormick, W. C., McCurry, S. M., Schellenberg, G. D., . . . Frölich, L. (1999). Impaired olfaction as a risk factor for cognitive decline: Interaction with Apolipoprotein E-04 status. *Neurology, 53,* 1480–1487.

Greenberg, D. A., Aminoff, M. J., & Simon, R. P. (2002). *Clinical Neurology* (5th ed.). New York, NY: Lange Medical Books/McGraw-Hill.

Grisso, T., & Appelbaum, P. (1998). *Assessing competence to consent and treatment: A guide for physicians and other health professionals.* New York, NY: Oxford University Press.

Hall, G. R. (1994). Caring for people with Alzheimer's disease using the conceptual model of progressively lowered stress threshold in the clinical setting. *The Nursing Clinics of North America, 29,* 129–141.

Hall, G. R., & Buckwalter, K. C. (1987). Progressively lowered stress threshold: A conceptual model for care of adults with Alzheimer's disease. *Archives of Psychiatric Nursing, 1*(6), 399–406.

Hamilton, M. (1959). The assessment of anxiety states by rating. *The British Journal of Medical Psychology, 32,* 50–55.

Hamilton, M. (1960). A rating scale for depression. *Journal of Neurology, Neurosurgery, and Psychiatry, 23,* 56–62. doi:10.1136/jnnp.23.1.56

Harper, D. G., Volicer, L., Stopa, E. G., McKee, A. C., Nitta, M., & Satlin, A. (2005). Disturbance of endogenous circadian rhythm in aging and Alzheimer disease. *The American Journal of Geriatric Psychiatry, 13,* 359–368.

Harris, R. (2009). *ACT with love: Stop struggling, reconcile differences, and strengthen your relationship with acceptance and commitment therapy.* Oakland, CA: New Harbinger Publications.

Hatfield, C. F., Herbert, J., van Someren, E. J., Hodges, J. R., & Hastings, M. H. (2004). Disrupted daily activity/rest cycles in relation to daily cortisol rhythms of home-dwelling patients with early Alzheimer's dementia. *Brain, 127,* 1061–1074. doi:10.1093/brain/awh129

Hayes, S. C., Hayes, L. J., Reese, H. W., & Sarbin, T. R. (Eds.). (1993). *Varieties of scientific contextualism.* Reno, NV: Context Press.

Hayes, S. C., Luoma, J. B., Bond, F. W., Masuda, A., & Lillis, J. (2006). Acceptance and commitment therapy: Model, processes, and outcomes. *Behaviour Research and Therapy, 44,* 1–25. doi:10.1016/j.brat.2005.06.006

Hayes, S. C., Masuda, A., Bissett, R., Luoma, J., & Guerrero, L. F. (2004). DBT, FAR, and ACT: How empirically oriented are the new behavior therapy technologies? *Behavior Therapy, 35,* 35–54. doi:10.1016/S0005-7894(04)80003-0

Hayes, S. C., Strosahl, K. D., & Wilson, K. G. (1999). *Acceptance and commitment therapy: An experiential approach to behavior change.* New York, NY: Guilford Press.

Hefferline, R. F., & Perrera, T. B. (1963, March). Proprioceptive discrimination of a covert operant without its observation by the subject. *Science, 139,* 834–835. doi:10.1126/science.139.3557.834

Hinrichsen, G. A., & Niederehe, G. (1994). Dementia management strategies and adjustment of family members of older patients. *The Gerontologist, 34,* 95–102.

Hoffman, D. (Producer & Director). (1994). *Complaints of a dutiful daughter* [Motion picture]. USA: Women Make Movies.

Holsinger, T., Deveau, J., Boustani, M., & Williams, J. W. (2007). Does this patient have dementia? *JAMA, 297,* 2391–2404. doi:10.1001/jama.297.21.2391

Horn, S. D., Bender, S. A., Bergstrom, N., Cook, A. S., Ferguson, M. L., Rimmasch, H. L., . . . Voss, A. C. (2002). Description of the National Pressure Ulcer Long-

Term Care Study. *Journal of the American Geriatrics Society, 50,* 1816–1825. doi:10.1046/j.1532-5415.2002.50510.x

Hoyer, W. J., Mishara, B. L., & Riebel, R. G. (1975). Problem behaviors as operants: Applications with elderly individuals. *The Gerontologist, 15,* 452–456.

Hubbard, G., Cook, A., Tester, S., & Downs, M. (2002). Beyond words: Older people with dementia using and interpreting nonverbal behavior. *Journal of Aging Studies, 16,* 155–167. doi:10.1016/S0890-4065(02)00041-5

Hughes, C. P., Berg, L., Danziger, W. L., Coben, L. A., & Martin, R. L. (1982). A new clinical scale for the staging of dementia. *The British Journal of Psychiatry, 140,* 566–572. doi:10.1192/bjp.140.6.566

Hussian, R. A. (1981). *Geriatric psychology: A behavioral perspective.* New York, NY: Van Nostrand Reinhold.

Hutchinson, A. D., & Mathias, J. L. (2007). Neuropsychological deficits in fronto-temporal dementia and Alzheimer's disease: A meta-analytic review. *Journal of Neurology, Neurosurgery, and Psychiatry, 78,* 917–928. doi:10.1136/jnnp.2006.100669

Inouye, S. K., & Ferrucci, L. (2006). Elucidating the pathophysiology of delirium and the interrelationship of delirium and dementia. *Journal of Gerontology: Medical Sciences, 61A,* 1277–1280.

Jacobson, N. S., & Margolin, G. (1979). *Marital therapy: Strategies based on social learning and behavioral exchange principles.* New York, NY: Brunner/Mazel.

Janevic, M. J., & Connell, C. M. (2004). Exploring self-care among dementia caregivers: The role of perceived support in accomplishing exercise goals. *Journal of Women & Aging, 16,* 71–86. doi:10.1300/J074v16n01_06

Johns, M. W. (1991). A new method for measuring daytime sleepiness: The Epworth Sleepiness Scale. *Sleep, 14,* 540–545.

Jurica, P. J., Leitten, C. L., & Mattis, S. (2002). *Dementia Rating Scale-2 (DRS-2) professional manual.* Odessa, FL: Psychological Assessment Resources.

Karlawish, J. (2008). Measuring decision-making capacity in cognitively impaired individuals. *Neuro-Signals, 16,* 91–98. doi:10.1159/000109763

Katzman, R. (2002). Diagnosis and management of dementia. In R. Katzman & J. W. Rowe (Eds.), *Principles of geriatric neurology* (pp. 167–206). Philadelphia, PA: F. A. Davis.

Kaufman, D. W., Kelly, J. P., Rosenberg, L., Anderson, T. E., & Mitchell, A. A. (2002). Recent patterns of medication use in the ambulatory adult population of the United States: The Slone Survey. *JAMA, 287,* 337–344. doi:10.1001/jama.287.3.337

Kim, S. Y., Kim, H. M., Langa, K. M., Karlawish, J. H., Knopman, D. S., & Appelbaum, P. S. (2009). Surrogate consent for dementia research: A national survey of older Americans. *Neurology, 72,* 149–155. doi:10.1212/01.wnl.0000339039.18931.a2

King, A. C., Baumann, K., O'Sullivan, P., Wilcox, S., & Castro, C. (2002). Effects of moderate-intensity exercise on physiological, behavioral, and emotional responses to family caregiving: A randomized controlled trial. *Journal of Gerontology: Medical Sciences, 57*(1), M26–M36.

Kolanowski, A. M., Litaker, M., & Buettner, L. (2005). Efficacy of theory-based activities for behavioral symptoms of dementia. *Nursing Research, 54*(4), 219–228. doi:10.1097/00006199-200507000-00003

Kovach, C. R., Noonan, P. E., Schlidt, A. M., & Wells, T. (2005). A model of consequences of need-driven, dementia-compromised behavior. *Journal of Nursing Scholarship, 37*(2), 134–140. doi:10.1111/j.1547-5069.2005.00025_1.x

Kukull, W. A., & Bowen, J. D. (2009). Public health, epidemiology, and neurologic diseases. In R. Detels, J. McEwen, R. Beaglehole, & H. Tanaka (Eds.), *Oxford textbook of public health: The practice of public health* (5th ed., Vol. 3, pp. 1132–1159). Oxford, England: Oxford University Press.

Kukull, W. A., Brenner, D. E., Speck, C. E., Nochlin, D., Bowen, J., McCormick, W., . . . Larson, E. B. (1994). Causes of death associated with Alzheimer disease: Variation by level of cognitive impairment before death. *Journal of the American Geriatrics Society, 42*, 723–726.

Kurz, A. F., & Lautenschlager, N. T. (2010). The concept of dementia: Retain, reframe, rename or replace? *International Psychogeriatrics, 22*, 37–42. doi:10.1017/S1041610209991013

Lawton, M. P. (1974). Social ecology and the health of older people. *American Journal of Public Health, 64*, 257–260. doi:10.2105/AJPH.64.3.257

Lawton, M. P. (1991). A multidimensional view of quality of life in frail elders. In J. E. Birren, J. E. Lubben, J. C. Rowe, & D. E. Deutchman (Eds.), *The concept and measurement of quality of life in the frail elderly* (pp. 3–27). San Diego, CA: Academic Press.

Lawton, M. P., & Brody, E. M. (1969). Assessment of older people: Self-maintaining and instrumental activities of daily living. *The Gerontologist, 9*, 179–186.

Lecouturier, J., Bamford, C., Hughes, J. C., Francis, J. J., Foy, R., Johnston, M., & Eccles, M. P. (2008). Appropriate disclosure of a diagnosis of dementia: Identifying the key behaviors of "best practice." *BMC Health Services Research, 8*, 95. doi:10.1186/1472-6963-8-95

Lee, J. H., Friedland, R., Whitehouse, P. J., & Woo, J. I. (2004). Twenty-four-hour rhythms of sleep–wake cycle and temperature in Alzheimer's disease. *The Journal of Neuropsychiatry and Clinical Neurosciences, 16*, 192–198. doi:10.1176/appi.neuropsych.16.2.192

Lewinsohn, P. M., Antonuccio, D. O., Steinmetz, J., & Teri, L. (1984). *The Coping with Depression Course*. Eugene, OR: Castalia Publishing.

Lewinsohn, P. M., & Graf, M. (1973). Pleasant activities and depression. *Journal of Consulting and Clinical Psychology, 41*, 261–268. doi:10.1037/h0035142

Lewinsohn, P. M., Muñoz, R. F., Youngren, M. A., & Zeiss, A. M. (1992). *Control your depression*. New York, NY: Fireside Books.

Lewis, J. J. (2009). Dorothy Parker quotes. *About.com: Women's history*. Retrieved from http://womenshistory.about.com/od/quotes/a/dorothy_parker.htm

Lezak, M. D. (1995). *Neuropsychological assessment* (3rd ed.). New York, NY: Oxford University Press.

Lindau, S. T., Schumm, L. P., Laumann, E. O., Levinson, W., O'Muircheartaigh, C. A., & Waite, L. J. (2007). A study of sexuality and health among older adults in the United States. *The New England Journal of Medicine, 357*(8), 762–774. doi:10.1056/NEJMoa067423

Lindsey, P. L., & Buckwalter, K. C. (2009). Psychotic events in Alzheimer's disease: Application of the PLST model. *Journal of Gerontological Nursing, 35*(8), 20–27. doi:10.3928/00989134-20090706-05

Loewenstein, D. A., Amigo, E., Duara, R., Guterman, A., Hurwitz, D., Berkowitz, N., . . . Wilkie, F. (1989). A new scale for the assessment of functional status in Alzheimer's disease and related disorders. *Journal of Gerontology: Psychological Sciences, 44*(4), 114–121.

Logsdon, R. G., Gibbons, L. E., McCurry, S. M., & Teri, L. (1999). Quality of life in Alzheimer's disease: Patient and caregiver reports. *Journal of Mental Health and Aging, 5*, 21–32.

Logsdon, R. G., Gibbons, L. E., McCurry, S. M., & Teri, L. (2002). Assessing quality of life in older adults with cognitive impairment. *Psychosomatic Medicine, 64*, 510–519.

Logsdon, R. G., McCurry, S. M., & Teri, L. (2007). Evidence-based psychological treatments for disruptive behaviors in individuals with dementia. *Psychology and Aging, 22*, 28–36. doi:10.1037/0882-7974.22.1.28

Logsdon, R. G., Pike, K. C., McCurry, S. M., Hunter, P., Maher, J., Snyder, L., & Teri, L.. (2010). Early stage memory loss support groups: Outcomes from a randomized controlled clinical trial. *Journals of Gerontology. Series B: Psychological Sciences and Social Sciences*.

Logsdon, R. G., Teri, L., Weiner, M. F., Gibbons, L. E., Raskind, M., Peskinds, E., Thal, L. J. (1999). Assessment of agitation in Alzheimer's disease: The Agitated Behavior in Dementia scale. *Journal of the American Geriatrics Society, 47*, 1354–1358.

Lütz, M. (2009). *Irre! Wir behandeln die falschen: Unser Problem sind die Normalen— eine heitere Seelenkunde* [Way off! We're treating the wrong ones: Normality is our problem—playful soul-searching by a psychiatrist]. Güterslohe, Germany: Gütersloher Verlagshaus.

Lyketsos, C. G., Colenda, C. C., Beck, C., Blank, K., Doraiswamy, M. P., Kalunian, D. A., & Yaffe, K. (2006). Position statement of the American Association for Geriatric Psychiatry regarding principles of care for patients with dementia resulting from Alzheimer disease. *The American Journal of Geriatric Psychiatry, 14*, 561–573. doi:10.1097/01.JGP.0000221334.65330.55

Lyketsos, C. G., Lopez, O., Jones, B., Fitzpatrick, A., Breitner, J., & DeKosky, S. (2002). Prevalence of neuropsychiatric symptoms in dementia and mild cognitive impairment: Results from the cardiovascular health study. *JAMA, 288,* 1475–1483. doi:10.1001/jama.288.12.1475

Madhusoodanan, S., Shah, P., Brenner, R., & Gupta, S. (2007). Pharmacological treatment of the psychosis of Alzheimer's disease: What is the best approach? [Review]. *CNS Drugs, 21,* 101–115. doi:10.2165/00023210-200721020-00002

Martell, C., Addis, M. E., & Jacobson, N. S. (2001). *Depression in context: Strategies for guided action.* New York, NY: Norton.

Martin, J. L., & Ancoli-Israel, S. (2008). Sleep disturbances in long-term care. *Clinics in Geriatric Medicine, 24,* 39–50. doi.org/10.1016/j.cger.2007.08.001

McCurry, S. M. (2006). *When a family member has dementia: Steps to becoming a resilient caregiver.* Westport, CT: Praeger.

McCurry, S. M., Gibbons, L. E., Logsdon, R. G., Vitiello, M. V., & Teri, L. (2005). Nighttime insomnia treatment and education for Alzheimer's disease: A randomized, controlled trial. *Journal of the American Geriatrics Society, 53,* 793–802. doi:10.1111/j.1532-5415.2005.53252.x

McCurry, S. M., Gibbons, L. E., Logsdon, R. G., Vitiello, M. V., & Teri, L. (2009). Insomnia in caregivers of persons with dementia: Who is at risk and what can be done about it? *Sleep Medicine Clinics, 4,* 519–526. doi:10.1016/j.jsmc.2009.07.005

McCurry, S. M., LaFazia, D. M., Pike, K. C., Logsdon, R. G., & Teri, L. (2009). Managing sleep disturbances in adult family homes: Recruitment and implementation of a behavioral treatment program. *Geriatric Nursing, 30,* 36–44. doi:10.1016/j.gerinurse.2008.05.001

McCurry, S. M., Logsdon, R. G., Teri, L., & Vitiello, M. V. (2007). Sleep disturbances in caregivers of persons with dementia: Contributing factors and treatment implications. *Sleep Medicine Reviews, 11,* 143–153. doi:10.1016/j.smrv.2006.09.002

McCurry, S. M., Reynolds, C. F., Ancoli-Israel, S., Teri, L., & Vitiello, M. V. (2000). Treatment of sleep disturbance in Alzheimer's disease. *Sleep Medicine Reviews, 4,* 603–628. doi:10.1053/smrv.2000.0127

McKim, W. A. (2003). *Drugs and behavior: An introduction to behavioral pharmacology* (5th ed.). Upper Saddle River, NJ: Pearson Education.

Meeks, T. W., & Jeste, D. V. (2008). Beyond the black box: What is the role for antipsychotics in dementia? *Current Psychiatry, 7*(6), 50–65.

Miller, R. S., & Lefcourt, H. M. (1982). The assessment of social intimacy. *Journal of Personality Assessment, 46,* 514–518. doi:10.1207/s15327752jpa4605_12

Mitchell, A. J. (2009). A meta-analysis of the accuracy of the Mini-Mental State Examination in the detection of dementia and mild cognitive impairment. *Journal of Psychiatric Research, 43,* 411–431. doi:10.1016/j.jpsychires.2008.04.014

Mitchell, P. H., Veith, R. C., Becker, K. J., Buzaitis, A., Cain, K. C., Fruin, M., . . . Teri, L. (2009). Brief psychosocial–behavioral intervention with antidepressant reduces poststroke depression significantly more than usual care with antidepressant. Living well with stroke: Randomized, controlled trial. *Stroke, 40,* 3073–3078. doi:10.1161/STROKEAHA.109.549808

Mossello, E., & Boncinelli, M. (2006). Mini-Mental State Examination: A 30-year story. *Aging: Clinical and Experimental Research, 18*(4), 271–273.

Müller, G., Richter, R. A., Weisbrod, S., & Klingberg, F. (1992). Impaired tactile pattern recognition in the early stage of primary degenerative dementia compared with normal aging. *Archives of Gerontology and Geriatrics, 14*(3), 215–225. doi:10.1016/0167-4943(92)90022-V

National Institute on Aging. (2010). *Home safety for people with Alzheimer's disease* (NIH Publication No. 02-5179). Silver Spring, MD: Alzheimer's Disease Education and Referral (ADEAR) Center.

Omnibus Budget Reconciliation Act, 42 C.F.R. § 483.25 (1987).

Osler, W. (1932). *Aequanimitas* (3rd rev. ed.). New York, NY: McGraw-Hill.

Perrault, A., Oremus, M., Demers, L., Vida, S., & Wolfson, C. (2000). Review of outcome measurement instruments in Alzheimer's disease drug trials: Psychometric properties of behavior and mood scales. *Journal of Geriatric Psychiatry and Neurology, 13*(4), 181–196. doi:10.1177/089198870001300403

Pinker, S., & Bloom, P. (1990). Natural language and natural selection. *The Behavioral and Brain Sciences, 13,* 707–784.

Poling, A., & Byrne, T. (2000). *Introduction to behavioral pharmacology.* Reno, NV: Context Press.

Radloff, L. (1977). The CES-D Scale: A self-report depression scale for research in the general population. *Applied Psychological Measurement, 1,* 385–401. doi:10.1177/014662167700100306

Reifler, B. V., Larson, E. B., & Teri, L. (1987). An outpatient geriatric psychiatry assessment and treatment service. *Clinics in Geriatric Medicine, 3,* 203–209.

Reisberg, B., Borenstein, J., Salob, S. P., Ferris, S. H., Franssen, E., & Georgotas, A. (1987). Behavioral symptoms in Alzheimer's disease: Phenomenology and treatment. *The Journal of Clinical Psychiatry, 48*(Suppl. 5), 9–15.

Reiss, S., & Aman, M. G. (Eds.). (1998). *Psychotropic medications and developmental disabilities: The international consensus handbook.* Columbus, OH: The Ohio State University Nisonger Center.

Rizzo, M., Anderson, S. W., Dawson, J., & Nawrot, M. (2000). Vision and cognition in Alzheimer's disease. *Neuropsychologia, 38,* 1157–1169. doi:10.1016/S0028-3932(00)00023-3

Roberts, M. (1996). *The man who listens to horses.* New York, NY: Random House.

Robinson, B. (1983). Validation of a Caregiver Strain Index. *Journals of Gerontology, 38*(3), 344–348.

Robinson-Whelen, S., Tada, Y., MacCallum, R. C., McGuire, L., & Kiecolt-Glaser, J. K. (2001). Long-term caregiving: What happens when it ends? *Journal of Abnormal Psychology, 110,* 573–584. doi:10.1037/0021-843X.110.4.573

Rosen, W. G., Mohs, R. C., & Davis, K. L. (1984). A new rating scale for Alzheimer's disease. *The American Journal of Psychiatry, 141,* 1356–1364.

Rosenberg, F. (2009). The MoMA Alzheimer's Project: Programming and resources for making art accessible to people with Alzheimer's disease and their caregivers. *Arts and Health, 1,* 93–97. doi:10.1080/17533010802528108

Ross, G. W., & Bowen, J. D. (2002). The diagnosis and differential diagnosis of dementia. *The Medical Clinics of North America, 86,* 455–476. doi:10.1016/S0025-7125(02)00009-3

Royall, D. R., Cordes, J. A., & Polk, M. (1998). CLOX: An executive clock drawing task. *Journal of Neurology, Neurosurgery, and Psychiatry, 64,* 588–594. doi:10.1136/jnnp.64.5.588

Royall, D. R., Mahurin, R. K., & Gray, K. F. (1992). Bedside assessment of executive cognitive impairment: The executive interview. *Journal of the American Geriatrics Society, 40,* 1221–1226.

Russo, J., & Vitaliano, P. P. (1995). Life events as correlates of burden in spouse caregivers of persons with Alzheimer's disease. *Experimental Aging Research, 21,* 273–294. doi:10.1080/03610739508253985

Sack, R. L., Auckley, D., Auger, R. R., Carskadon, M. A., Wright, K. P., Vitiello, M. V., & Zhdanova, I. V. (2007). Circadian rhythm sleep disorders: Part II. Advanced sleep phase disorder, delayed sleep phase disorder, free-running disorder, and irregular sleep–wake rhythm. An American Academy of Sleep Medicine review. *Sleep, 30,* 1484–1501.

Salva, A., Coll-Planas, L., Bruce, S., De Groot, L., Andrieu, S., Abellan, G., . . . The Task Force on Nutrition and Ageing of the IAGG and the IANA. (2009). Nutritional assessment of residents in long-term care facilities (LTCFs): Recommendations of the Task Force on Nutrition and Ageing of the IAGG European Region and the IANA. *The Journal of Nutrition, Health & Aging, 13*(6), 475–483. doi:10.1007/s12603-009-0097-7

Salzman, C. (Ed.). (2005). *Clinical geriatric psychopharmacology* (4th ed.). New York, NY: Lippincott Williams & Wilkins.

Schulz, R., & Martire, L. M. (2004). Family caregiving of persons with dementia: Prevalence, health effects, and support strategies. *The American Journal of Geriatric Psychiatry, 12,* 240–249. doi:10.1176/appi.ajgp.12.3.240

Schulz, R., Newsom, J. T., Mittlemark, M., Burton, L. C., Hirsh, C., & Jackson, S. (1997). Health effects of caregiving: The Caregiver Health Effects Study. *Annals of Behavioral Medicine, 19,* 110–116. doi:10.1007/BF02883327

Schulz, R., O'Brien, A., Bookwala, J., & Fleissner, K. (1995). Psychiatric and physical morbidity effects of dementia caregiving: Prevalence, correlates, and causes. *The Gerontologist, 35,* 771–791.

Schulz, R., O'Brien, A., Czaja, S., Ory, M., Norris, R., Martire, L. M., . . . Stevens, A. (2002). Dementia caregiver intervention research: In search of clinical significance. *The Gerontologist, 42*, 589–602.

Schulz, R., & Sherwood, P. R. (2008). Physical and mental health effects of family caregiving. *The American Journal of Nursing, 108*(9, Suppl), 23–27.

Selwood, A., Cooper, C., Owens, C., Blanchard, M., & Livingston, G. (2009). What would help me stop abusing? The family carer's perspective. *International Psychogeriatrics, 21*, 309–313. doi:10.1017/S104161020800834X

Shankar, K. K., Walker, M., Frost, D., & Orrell, M. W. (1999). The development of a valid and reliable scale for rating anxiety in dementia (RAID). *Aging & Mental Health, 3*, 39–49. doi:10.1080/13607869956424

Sikkes, S. A., de Lange-de Klerk, E. S., Pijnenburg, Y. A., Scheltens, P., & Uitdehaag, B. M. (2009). A systematic review of instrumental activities of daily living scales in dementia: Room for improvement. *Journal of Neurology, Neurosurgery, and Psychiatry, 80*, 7–12. doi:10.1136/jnnp.2008.155838

Sink, K. M., Holden, K. F., & Yaffe, K. (2005). Pharmacological treatment of neuropsychiatric symptoms of dementia: A review of the evidence. *JAMA, 293*, 596–608. doi:10.1001/jama.293.5.596

Skinner, H. A., Steinhauer, P. D., & Santa-Barbara, J. (1983). The Family Assessment Measure. *Canadian Journal of Community Mental Health, 2*, 91–105.

Small, G. W., Rabins, P. V., Barry, P. P., Buckholtz, N. S., DeKosky, S. T., Ferris, S. H., . . . Tune, L. E. (1997). Diagnosis and treatment of Alzheimer disease and related disorders. Consensus statement of the American Association for Geriatric Psychiatry, the Alzheimer's Association, and the American Geriatrics Society. *JAMA, 278*, 1363–1371. doi:10.1001/jama.278.16.1363

Smith, M., Gerdner, L. A., Hall, G. R., & Buckwalter, K. C. (2004). History, development, and future of the progressively lowered stress threshold: A conceptual model for dementia care. *Journal of the American Geriatrics Society, 52*, 1755–1760. doi:10.1111/j.1532-5415.2004.52473.x

Smith, M., Hall, G. R., Gerdner, L., & Buckwalter, K. C. (2006). Application of the progressively lowered stress threshold model across the continuum of care. *The Nursing Clinics of North America, 41*, 57–81. doi:10.1016/j.cnur.2005.09.006

Sohlberg, M. M., & Mateer, C. A. (2001). *Cognitive rehabilitation: An integrative neuropsychological approach.* New York, NY: Guilford Press.

Spreen, O., & Strauss, E. (1998). *A compendium of neuropsychological tests* (2nd ed.). New York, NY: Oxford University Press.

Steffen, A. M., McKibbin, C., Zeiss, A. M., Gallagher-Thompson, D., & Bandura, A. (2002). The Revised Scale for Caregiving Self-Efficacy: Reliability and validity studies. *Journal of Gerontology: Psychological Sciences, 57B*(1), 74–86.

Stolley, J. M., Reed, D., & Buckwalter, K. C. (2002). Caregiving appraisal and interventions based on the progressively lowered stress threshold model. *American*

Journal of Alzheimer's Disease and Other Dementias, 17(2), 110–120. doi:10.1177/153331750201700211

Strober, L. B., & Arnett, P. A. (2009). Assessment of depression in three medically ill, elderly populations: Alzheimer's disease, Parkinson's disease, and stroke. *The Clinical Neuropsychologist, 23,* 205–230. doi:10.1080/13854040802003299

Sunderland, T., Hill, J. L., Lawlor, B. A., & Molchan, S. E. (1988). NIMH Dementia Mood Assessment Scale (DMAS). *Psychopharmacology Bulletin, 24,* 747–751.

Tariot, P. N., Mack, J., Patterson, M., Edland, S. D., Weiner, M. F., Fillenbaum, G., . . . Stern, Y.. (1995). The CERAD Behavior Rating Scale for Dementia (BRSD). *The American Journal of Psychiatry, 152,* 1349–1357.

Teng, E. L., & Chui, H. C. (1987). The Modified Mini-Mental State (3MS) Examination. *The Journal of Clinical Psychiatry, 48,* 314–318.

Teng, E. L., Hasegawa, K., Homma, A., Imai, Y., Larson, E., Graves, A., . . . White, L. R. (1994). The Cognitive Abilities Screening Instrument (CASI): A practical test for cross-cultural epidemiological studies of dementia. *International Psychogeriatrics, 6,* 45–58. doi:10.1017/S1041610294001602

Teri, L. (1994). Behavioral treatment of depression in patients with dementia. *Alzheimer Disease and Associated Disorders, 8,* 66–74.

Teri, L., Gibbons, L. E., McCurry, S. M., Logsdon, R. G., Buchner, D. M., Barlow, W. E., . . . Larson, E. B. (2003). Exercise plus behavioral management in patients with Alzheimer disease: A randomized controlled trial. *JAMA, 290,* 2015–2022. doi:10.1001/jama.290.15.2015

Teri, L., Huda, P., Gibbons, L. E., Young, H., & van Leynseele, J. (2005). STAR: A dementia-specific training program for staff in assisted living residences. *The Gerontologist, 45,* 686–693.

Teri, L., & Logsdon, R. (1990). Assessment and management of behavioral disturbances in Alzheimer's disease. *Comprehensive Therapy, 16,* 36–42.

Teri, L., & Logsdon, R. G. (1991). Identifying pleasant activities for Alzheimer's disease patients: The Pleasant Events Schedule-AD. *The Gerontologist, 31,* 124–127.

Teri, L., & Logsdon, R. G. (1995). Methodologic issues regarding outcome measures for clinical drug trials of psychiatric complications in dementia. *Journal of Geriatric Psychiatry and Neurology, 8,* S8–S17. doi:10.1177/089198879500800103

Teri, L., Logsdon, R. G., & McCurry, S. M. (2005). The Seattle Protocols: Advances in behavioral treatment of Alzheimer's disease. In B. Vellas, L. J. Fitten, B. Winblad, H. Feldman, M. Grundman, & E. Giacobini (Eds.), *Research and practice in Alzheimer's disease and cognitive decline* (Vol. 10, pp. 153–158). Paris, France: Serdi Publisher.

Teri, L., Logsdon, R. G., & McCurry, S. M. (2008). Exercise interventions for dementia and cognitive impairment: The Seattle Protocols. *The Journal of Nutrition, Health & Aging, 12*(6), 391–394. doi:10.1007/BF02982672

Teri, L., Logsdon, R. G., Peskind, E., Raskind, M., Weiner, M. F., Tractenberg, R. E., ... Thal, L. J. (2000). Treatment of agitation in AD: A randomized, placebo-controlled clinical trial. *Neurology, 55*, 1271–1278.

Teri, L., Logsdon, R. G., Uomoto, J., & McCurry, S. (1997). Behavioral treatment of depression in dementia patients: A controlled clinical trial. *Journals of Gerontology: Series B, Psychological Sciences and Social Sciences, 52B*(4), P159–P166.

Teri, L., McCurry, S. M., Logsdon, R. G., & Gibbons, L. E. (2005). Training community consultants to help family members improve care: A randomized controlled trial. *The Gerontologist, 45*, 802–811.

Teri, L., McKenzie, G. L., LaFazia, D., Farran, C. J., Beck, C., Huda, P., ... Pike, K. C. (2009). Improving dementia care in assisted living residences: Staff responses to training. *Geriatric Nursing, 30*(3), 153–163. doi:10.1016/j.gerinurse.2008.07.002

Teri, L., McKenzie, G. L., Pike, K. C., Farran, C. J., Beck, C., Paun, O., & Lafazia, D. (2010). Staff training in assisted living: Evaluating treatment fidelity. *The American Journal of Geriatric Psychiatry, 18*, 502–509.

Teri, L., Truax, P., Logsdon, R. G., Uomoto, J., Zarit, S., & Vitaliano, P. P. (1992). Assessment of behavioral problems in dementia: The Revised Memory and Behavior Problems Checklist. *Psychology and Aging, 7*, 622–631. doi:10.1037/0882-7974.7.4.622

Terman, M. (2007). Evolving applications of light therapy. *Sleep Medicine Reviews, 11*, 497–507. doi:10.1016/j.smrv.2007.06.003

Thal, L. J. (1997). Development of the Alzheimer's Disease Cooperative Study. *International Journal of Geriatric Psychopharmacology, 1*, 6–9.

Tippett, W. J., & Sergio, L. E. (2006). Visuomotor integration is impaired in early stage Alzheimer's disease. *Brain Research, 1102*, 92–102. doi:10.1016/j.brainres.2006.04.049

Tombaugh, T. N., & McIntyre, N. J. (1992). The Mini-Mental State Examination: A comprehensive review. *Journal of the American Geriatrics Society, 40*, 922–935.

Tractenberg, R. E., Singer, C. M., Cummings, J. L., & Thal, L. J. (2003). The Sleep Disorders Inventory (SDI): An instrument for studies of sleep disturbance in persons with Alzheimer's disease. *Journal of Sleep Research, 12*, 331–337.

Tranel, D., & Damasio, A. (1985, June). Knowledge without awareness: An autonomic index of facial recognition by prosopagnosics. *Science, 228*, 1453–1454. doi:10.1126/science.4012303

Treatment of agitation in older persons with dementia. The Expert Consensus Panel for agitation in dementia. (1998, April). *Postgraduate Medicine, Spec No*, 1–88.

Ulrich, R. E., & Azrin, N. H. (1962). Reflexive fighting in response to aversive stimulation. *Journal of the Experimental Analysis of Behavior, 5*, 511–520.

U.S. Food and Drug Administration. (2009a). *Alert for health care professionals: Risperidone (marketed as Risperdal)*. Retrieved from http://www.fda.gov/Drugs/

DrugSafety/PostmarketDrugSafetyInformationforPatientsandProviders/ucm 152291.htm

U.S. Food and Drug Administration. (2009b). *Information for health care professionals: Conventional antipsychotics*. Retrieved from http://www.fda.gov/Drugs/DrugSafety/ PostmarketDrugSafetyInformationforPatientsandProviders/ucm124830.htm

Vernooij-Dassen, M. J., Feeling, A. J., Brummelkamp, E., Dauzenberg, M. G., van den Bos, G. A., & Grol, R. (1999). Assessment of caregiver's competence in dealing with the burden of caregiving for a dementia patient: A short sense of competence questionnaire (SSCQ) suitable for clinical practice. *Journal of the American Geriatrics Society, 47,* 256–257.

Vitaliano, P. P., Russo, J., Young, H. M., Becker, J., & Maiuro, R. D. (1991). The Screen for Caregiver Burden. *The Gerontologist, 31,* 76–83.

Vitaliano, P. P., Young, H. M., Russo, J., Romano, J., & Magana-Amato, A. (1993). Does expressed emotion in spouses predict subsequent problems among care recipients with Alzheimer's disease? *Journal of Gerontology: Psychological Sciences, 48*(4), 202–209.

Vitaliano, P. P., Zhang, J., & Scanlan, J. M. (2003). Is caregiving hazardous to ones physical health? A meta-analysis. *Psychological Bulletin, 129,* 946–972. doi:10.1037/ 0033-2909.129.6.946

Vitiello, M. V., & Borson, S. (2001). Sleep disturbances in patients with Alzheimer's disease: Epidemiology, pathophysiology and treatment. *CNS Drugs, 15,* 777–796. doi:10.2165/00023210-200115100-00004

Wagnild, G. M., & Young, H. M. (1993). Development and psychometric evaluation of the Resilience Scale. *Journal of Nursing Measurement, 1,* 165–178.

Wallace, M., & Safer, M. (2009). Hypersexuality among cognitively impaired older adults. *Geriatric Nursing, 30*(4), 230–237. doi:10.1016/j.gerinurse.2008.09.001

Ware, J. E., Snow, K. K., Kosinski, M., & Gandek, B. (1993). *SF-36 health survey. Manual and interpretation guide*. Boston, MA: Nimrod Press.

Watson, D., Clark, L. A., & Tellegen, A. (1988). Development and validation of brief measures of positive and negative affect: The PANAS scales. *Journal of Personality and Social Psychology, 54,* 1063–1070. doi:10.1037/0022-3514.54.6.1063

Wesolowski, M. D., & Zencius, A. H. (1994). *A practical guide to head injury rehabilitation: A focus on postacute residential treatment*. New York, NY: Plenum Press.

Whall, A. L., Colling, K. B., Kolanowski, A., Kim, H., Son Hong, G. R., DeCicco, B., . . . Beck, C. (2008). Factors associated with aggressive behavior among nursing home residents with dementia. *The Gerontologist, 48,* 721–731.

Whall, A. L., & Kolanowski, A. M. (2004). The need-driven dementia-compromised behavior model—A framework for understanding the behavioral symptoms of dementia. *Aging & Mental Health, 8*(2), 106–108. doi:10.1080/1360786041000 1649590

Woods, D. L., Rapp, C. G., & Beck, C. (2004). Escalation/de-escalation patterns of behavioral symptoms of persons with dementia. *Aging & Mental Health, 8*(2), 126–132. doi:10.1080/13607860410001649635

Yesavage, J., Brink, T., Rose, T., Lum, O., Huang, V., Adey, M., & Leirer, V. O. (1983). Development and validation of a geriatric depression screening scale: A preliminary report. *Journal of Psychiatric Research*, *17*, 37–49. doi:10.1016/0022-3956(82)90033-4

Zarit, S. H., Todd, P. A., & Zarit, J. M. (1986). Subjective burden of husbands and wives as caregivers: A longitudinal study. *The Gerontologist*, *26*, 260–266.

Zarit, S. H., & Femia, E. E. (2008). A future for family care and dementia intervention research? Challenges and strategies. *Aging & Mental Health*, *12*(1), 5–13. doi:10.1080/13607860701616317

Zettle, R. (2007). *ACT for depression: A clinician's guide to using acceptance and commitment therapy in treating depression*. Oakland, CA: New Harbinger Publications.

INDEX

Ameliorate excess disability, *continued*
    and depression, 42, 85
    description of, 42–43
    long-term relationships case example,
        95–96
    and medical comorbidities, 67–69
    and medical illness, 42, 81–85
    role identities case example, 48
    and sensory loss, 42, 74–76
    severe impairment case example, 83
    and sleep disturbances, 71–72
American Association for Retired
        Persons (AARP), 173
American Health Assistance Foundation
        (AHAF), 173
Antecedents, 28, 119n9
Antipsychotic medications, 77
Anxiety, 42, 114–116
Anxiolytic drugs, 106n2, 119n9
Apathy, 20
Aphasia, 16
Appelbaum, P., 61
Apraxia, 16
Area Agencies on Aging (AAA), 173
Arguments, 41, 127
Arts for the Aging Project, 134
Assessment measures, 155–157
Attention difficulties, 18
Attorneys-in-fact, 62, 63

Baseline activity level, 73
Bechara, A., 15n4
Behavioral changes, 20–21, 109–130
    with aggression, 120–121
    alternative therapies for, 130
    A • B • Cs of, 26–33
    and circadian rhythm disturbances,
        121–122
    and consequences in context, 118–120
    and disorders, 12–16
    with erroneous beliefs and accusatory
        behavior, 125–130
    nonpharmacological solutions for,
        110–113
    personal context of, 24
    specific behavior challenges with,
        113–118
    and stressors in A • B • C model,
        123–124
    with wandering behaviors, 121–122,
        124–125

Behavioral strengths, 166
Behavior analysis, 24
Behaviorism, radical, 26n3
Behavior management interventions, 111
Behaviors. *See also* Behavioral changes
    accusatory and threatening,
        162–163, 169
    of caregiver, 167–168
    consequences as shapers of, 32–33
    and contextual model, 113–118
    descriptions of, 27
    fearful and self-protective, 162, 169
    functional analysis of, 34–36
    labeled as problematic, 132
    positive reinforcement of, 29–32
    principles for analysis of, 25–26
    punishment for, 30–32
    in sample consultation report, 165,
        168–169
    screening instruments for, 156–157
    self-protective, 101–102
    shaped by contingencies, 32–33
Bell, V., 24
*The Best Friends Approach to Dementia
        Care* (V. Bell & D. Troxel), 24
Blame, 94
Boustani, M., 11
Bowel functioning, 72–73
Bowen, J. D., 11
Brain pathology, 10, 11
Brain tumors, 13
Buckwalter, K. C., 122n11
Burgio, L. D., 26n3
Burnout, 140–141
Byrne, T., 119n9

Cancer, 13
Cardiogenic dementia, 13
Caregivers
    depression in, 114, 115, 139n5
    health problems of, 139–140
    instrumental tasks and skills of,
        167–168
    in meaningful activities, 135–136
    medical status of, 167
    mood, affect, and behavior of, 167–168
    and motivational changes, 20
    problem-solving strategies for, 92–94
    professional, 102
    quality of life for, 138–143

ABOUT THE AUTHORS

Susan M. McCurry, PhD, is research professor in the University of Washington Department of Psychosocial and Community Health and adjunct research professor in psychiatry and behavioral sciences. She is a clinical psychologist specializing in gerontology and has worked with older adults with memory loss and their families for over 20 years. She is a fellow in the Gerontological Society of America, and has coauthored over 100 professional publications and book chapters. Her ongoing clinical research focuses on (a) assessment and treatment of sleep disturbances in older adults with dementia or other co-morbid medical conditions such as chronic pain; (b) development and evaluation of training programs for family and professional staff caring for persons with dementia; and (c) examination of the environmental, behavioral, and psychosocial factors associated with cognitive decline. She is author of the book *When a Family Member Has Dementia: Steps to Becoming a Resilient Caregiver* (2006), a practical and positive guide for family and professional caregivers of persons with dementia.

Claudia Drossel, PhD, received her PhD in experimental psychology in 2004 from Temple University, with a specialization in the organization of learning as well as functional and contextual approaches to affect, behavior, and cognition. She currently is a doctoral candidate in the University of Nevada, Reno's clinical gerontology program, where she focuses on researching, practicing, and disseminating the contextual approach to dementia care. From 2005 through 2010, Dr. Drossel was associate director of the Nevada Caregiver Support Center, a state-funded, evidence-based, consumer-directed service program for individuals with dementia and their families, recognized in June 2008 by the U.S. Administration on Aging as a Program Champion. Dr. Drossel has developed and conducted statewide professional training for dementia care providers and has implemented group interventions for family caregivers to remove barriers to evidence-based dementia care practices. She has also coauthored geropsychological and general publications on contextual approaches to behavior.